Teaching the Practitioners of Care

Interpretive Studies in Healthcare and the Human Sciences

VOLUME 2

Teaching the Practitioners of Care

New Pedagogies for the Health Professions

Nancy L. Diekelmann

Volume Editor

THE UNIVERSITY OF WISCONSIN PRESS

To John Diekelmann and Jay Ironside,

our life partners in scholarship,

for their collaboration and love.

The University of Wisconsin Press
1930 Monroe Street
Madison, Wisconsin 53711

www.wisc.edu/wisconsinpress/

3 Henrietta Street
London WC2E 8LU, England

5   4   3   2   1

Printed in the United States of America

Library of Congress Cataloging-in-Publication Data

Teaching the practitioners of care : new pedagogies for the health professions / Nancy L. Diekelmann, volume editor.
    p. ; cm. — (Interpretive studies in healthcare and the human sciences ; v. 2)
Includes bibliographical references and index.
    ISBN 0-299-18480-3 (cloth : alk. paper) — ISBN 0-299-18484-6 (paper : alk. paper)
    1. Nursing—Study and teaching.
    [DNLM: 1. Education, Nursing—methods, United States.   2. Teaching methods—
United States.   3. Nursing Research—United States. WY 18 T2535 2003]   I. Title:
Teaching the practitioners of care.   II. Diekelmann, Nancy L.   III. Series.
    RT71 .T347 2003
    610.73′071—dc21

                                                                                    2002014490

Contents

Teaching the Practitioners of Care

Introduction

Nancy L. Diekelmann, Pamela M. Ironside,
and Morgan Harlow

Do faculty in the health professions, even as they support the need to imple-
ment innovation and reform, continue to teach as they were taught and for a
healthcare system that no longer exists?

A rapidly changing healthcare system, the shift to community-based
care, and increasing diversity in student populations are challenging
health professions schools. Yet curricula in many of these schools continue to reflect the assumptions of hospital-based practice, merely adding clinical experience in community settings. The industrialization of
healthcare and the explosion of bioscience technologies call for a change
in the way health professionals practice, and consequently in the way
they are taught (Eitel, Kanz, Hortig, & Tesche, 2000; Jones, McArdle, &
O'Neill, 2002; Kassebaum & Cutler, 1998; Shatzer, 1998). But how do
teachers teach to a healthcare system in persistent transition? What possibilities exist for substantive reform?

*Teaching the Practitioners of Care: New Pedagogies for the Health
Professions* gathers interpretive, educational research in the health professions to complement the current reform in conventional approaches.
This gathering is not an attempt to devalue conventional pedagogy (outcomes education) in order to create a place for new approaches to health
professions education. Rather, the interpretive pedagogies *co-occur*

3

with other approaches, *including* conventional pedagogies. The studies in this book provide evidence and insights upon which teachers can initiate educational research and reform in their own classrooms and clinical settings. At a time when interpretive pedagogies are being developed in every discipline (Armstrong & Koffman, 2000; Berger & Ai, 2000; Kassebaum & Cutler, 1998; Neistadt, 1999), and there are calls for reform in medical education, pharmacy, and nursing (Fox, 1999; Iglehart, 2000; Lesky & Yonke, 2001) the voices gathered together in this second volume of the book series *Interpretive Studies in Healthcare and the Human Sciences* are timely and originary in bringing to the health professions *substantively new pedagogies* for transforming extant curricula. Herein are the insights of teacher-scholars who are developing and evaluating the new pedagogies in their teaching practice.

Toward Pedagogical Literacy

The need for faculty members to increase their pedagogical literacy has never been greater. Students in nursing often describe experiences that indicate they are "on strike," as evidenced by their use of resistance, silence, nonperformance, lateness, and absence (Diekelmann, 1991). According to Shor (1986), students resist any process that disempowers them and denies subjects important to them. Even as faculty members acknowledge these problems, as many are doing, teachers continue to teach as they were taught. This is in large part because faculty skills and pedagogical literacy are at a critically low level.

Furthermore, across the nation there is a serious and growing shortage of nursing faculty (DeYoung & Bliss, 1995; Post & Louden, 1997); it is expected that approximately one third of current faculty will retire between 1992 and 2006 (Plater, 1995; Post, 1997; Ryan & Irvine, 1994). No less significant is the ongoing problem of a shortage of nursing faculty educated as teachers (Princeton, 1992). Part-time and clinical adjunct faculty in nursing increasingly are providing instruction, even though most have not had preparation in teaching (DeSevo, 1995). These part-time and adjunct faculty have not had access to faculty development initiatives that emphasize knowledge, skills, and socialization to the role of nurse educator in order to adequately prepare students for changing healthcare environments (Benner, Hooper-Kyriakidis, & Stannard, 1999; Choudry, 1992; Diekelmann, 2001, 2002; DeSevo, 1995;

Norton & Spross, 1994; Opdycke, 1999; Sheehe & Schoener, 1994; Young, 1999). In graduate nursing programs emphasis is placed on research and the preparation of doctoral students, often to the exclusion of teacher preparation coursework and practica (American Association of Colleges of Nursing, 1995). Many disciplines believe that winging it for a semester or two as a teaching assistant is all the preparation a person needs in order to go on to teach the discipline. Likewise, teacher preparation coursework is often nonexistent in many health professions graduate curricula.

At precisely the time when health professions faculty most need to increase their pedagogical literacy and expand their teaching skills to respond to the challenges of contemporary teaching and healthcare environments, funding for faculty development is declining. Without substantive reform, however, the quality of health professions education for students will be at increased risk for failure.

Creating Student-Centered Pedagogies

A revolution is needed in nursing education no less dramatic than the one instigated by Florence Nightingale.

Sr. M. Mooney, personal communication, April 2000

We are supposed to be learning how to care for people . . . in a classroom where the students all fight over grades, and the teachers are defensive—ha! Walking the talk does matter. I think students and teachers could do a better job of caring despite our differences if we would put our minds to it.

Diekelmann, 2001

In general, there is more diversity in the health professions student population today. This population is older than it was 40 years ago, as people return to school to complete baccalaureate and graduate degrees, and it is increasingly common for students to already be in the workforce. Often they are caring for their own children, or for parents, and have little time to become involved in educational communities. Confronted with the immediacy of the need to work, they report high stress levels and concerns over the quality of their education and the abilities of schools to prepare them for future practice in healthcare (Boyer, 2000). Furthermore, the legacy of overreliance on teacher-centered pedagogies in the health professions has created learning climates that are competitive and isolating for students, teachers, and clinical preceptors. Paradoxically, while curricula espouse a commitment to developing interpersonal skills and the ability to work in groups, students are reporting that fear, anger, and anxiety characterize relationships with faculty.

In the health professions, students report feeling dependent on and controlled by faculty who on one hand keep them safe from making errors in clinical courses and on the other act as gatekeepers to the profession. Furthermore, *many faculty members are teaching a health-care system that no longer exists.* Even faculty in clinical courses report difficulty keeping up with changes in practice. Faculty who lecture rely on literature to keep them current, yet increasingly the changes are so rapid and profound that they report having trouble figuring out which changes to teach. Textbooks are out of date before they are published. The challenges of community-based care are slow to enter curricula other than through increased clinical time spent in the community. Teachers continue to teach an idealized care that is nonexistent and out of sync with the current healthcare system. A teacher describes her concern about the introductory course for beginning nursing students still teaching bedbaths:

Nurses DON'T give bedbaths and make beds anymore. They simply don't have time. Yet this continues to be the mainstay of our Fundamentals course . . . [When I challenged whether this skill needed to continue to be included] the argument from my colleagues . . . was that, "Yes, but this is when nurses can do their assessments and establish a relationship with the patient." Nerts!!!! Like as a professional RN you couldn't do a good assessment without giving a bath or establish a therapeutic relationship without scrubbing someone's backside. In fact, as a patient, if I'm having my backside scrubbed, I'm not all that into "therapeutic communication" with the scrubber! We simply have to look at all these carry-overs from our hospital-based curriculum. That healthcare system is just not here any more. Nurses need extraordinary observations skills in caring for increasingly more acutely ill patients . . . and they need very refined reflective . . . and contextual thinking skills that allow them to read the situations they confront all the while they work in a healthcare system that is increasingly community-based and in which they have fewer resources and DEFINITELY less support. We HAVE to change not only what but HOW we teach if we really want these students to be prepared!

How pedagogies both shape and are shaped by the phenomena they are developed to teach is an important discourse point in these studies. For example, how does a teacher-centered pedagogy reproduce power relationships within healthcare? Do caregivers have power and control over patients the way teachers have power and control over students? How does what (and how) we teach influence both the repertoire of skills obtained by students *and* how they see (and think about) their practice?

Are new partnerships among the healthcare professions needed? If so, then exploring how pedagogies encourage students to develop or discourage them from developing the skills of collaboration is crucial. For example, conventional pedagogy coursework often includes group projects that focus on developing collaborative and interpersonal skills in students with little attention paid to the ways they might use these skills in their classroom to influence the learning environment of the course. A teacher describes being aware of the dissonance created when the outcome of the assignment is achieved but the experiences of the students belie the outcome identified:

Yes [we assign students group projects], and when "group projects" don't work well . . . we make it the STUDENTS' problem. Like when one student is just along for the ride, then we put the responsibility on the other students to deal with the issue and [we forget] they are overwhelmed just getting the work done . . . and how many of them can't afford the possible "deduction in points" that are at risk by allowing a weak student to be involved in a meaningful way. So while we [teachers] USE group projects, we DON'T teach OR MODEL how to work as a community. We just think it will happen if we assign it.

Group work becomes a student learning assignment that is evaluated with little attention paid to how classroom environments teach (or fail to teach) students to become more expert in building communities (or groups) through developing collaborative interpersonal skills.

Interpretive Pedagogies in Higher Education

Although higher education has been dominated by conventional pedagogies, alternatives have been developed and have been shown to be effective (Barr & Tagg, 1995). These alternatives—critical, feminist, phenomenological, and postmodern pedagogies—are approaches to

learning, teaching, and schooling known collectively as interpretive pedagogies. Each shifts the focus from teacher-centered activities such as
lecturing and grading to community-oriented ones in which students
and teachers work together in learning. Although there are epistemological, theoretical, and practical differences between and among these
pedagogies, each assumes a "critical" position (Apple, 2001; Bromley &
Apple, 1998; Castells, et al., 1999; Giroux, 1997; Kerdeman, 1998;
Smith & Webster, 1997) and provides a way for teachers and students
to work together to critique and transform the learning process
(Ironside, 1997, 2001).

Teachers using critical and feminist pedagogies interpret the learning climate through the "lens" of democracy, empowerment, and social
action (Creager, Lunbeck, & Schiebinger, 2001; hooks, 2000; Kincheloe & Steinberg, 1998; Carlson & Apple, 1998), although teachers
ascribing to feminist pedagogies also make central how issues of gender
influence the learning climate (Donovan, 2001; Mayberry & Rose, 1999;
Cohee et al., 1998). For example, in a medical school in an all-school
meeting, the commitments of critical and feminist pedagogies emerged
in the discussion among teachers and students that focused on the issue
of how large auditoriums position teachers as speakers and students as
listeners. Students also questioned why women constituted less than
one-third of the faculty even though half the students in the department
were female. They questioned a recent curriculum change in which a
required course would only be taught once every four semesters. This
change would shift the course enrollment from 50 students per semester
to 200, perpetuating the use of an auditorium. In collaboration, teachers
and students decided not to change the curriculum and kept the classes
small, avoiding the distancing of teachers and promoting dialogue in
classes where teachers and students could better get to know and connect with one another.

Within postmodernism the focus is on challenging fundamental notions such as pedagogies themselves. And in critical postmodernism, the
self-evident or taken-for-granted assumptions in the practices of teaching and learning are deconstructed. One pharmacy school, for example,
discussed how unequal and devalued adjunct faculty felt because they
did not have a "legal" academic title even though they possessed the
skills, knowledge, and expertise needed to teach. The assumptions that
the teacher needs an academic title and/or one more degree than the

students were challenged, and faculty titles were given to all clinical teaching staff, including adjunct and instructional academic staff. The issue of labeling and degree preparation and how practices of controlling resources through labeling was deconstructed, and a series of titles based on expertise rather than degree preparation for all faculty evolved that was approved by the university. The use of interpretive pedagogies in the health professions is becoming more commonplace.

Interpretive Pedagogies in the Health Professions

Simply put, pedagogy is a particular approach to schooling, learning, and teaching. Embedded in each pedagogy are underlying assumptions and ways of seeing and thinking about the discipline—including considerations of what is taught, how it is taught, and what constitutes knowledge, knowing, learning, and being—as a nurse, physical therapist, or physician.

Phenomenological pedagogical research in the health professions has generated narratives of common experiences that show how students and teachers are using a variety of interpretive pedagogies seamlessly woven together to improve the learning climate for students (Andrews et al., 2001; Atwell-Vasey, 1998; Diekelmann, 2001; Diekelmann & Diekelmann, forthcoming; Haroutunian-Gordon, 1998; Hartrick, 2000; Hillocks, 1999; McEwan & Egan, 1995; Nehls, 1995; Noddings, 2002; van Manen, 1991). Strategies are aimed at increasing understanding among students and teachers through public storytelling and reflective thinking. For example, in one physical therapy class, students and teacher shared their perspectives on a class paper. Students requested that the three-page assignment be graded and returned during the next class meeting (two days later), but the teacher explained that he tried to give meaningful comments in response to each student's writing, and noted that, with 33 students in the class he would need as many as six hours to read the papers once and another three to six hours to write the comments. He then described the competing demands on his time in the next week, including his course load, committee work, and academic advising. Thus, the teacher exposed the tension between the demands of an academic role that made finding time to grade papers difficult and his desire to provide the students with meaningful feedback. The students discussed how immediate feedback allowed them to begin the next assignment early and how important "early starts" were to balancing their schedules. Students also shared what it was like for them to find time in their lives to do the assignments, to find baby sitters, to go to the library in the evenings and spend forty-five minutes trying to park in a safe area. The teacher's understanding of the meaning of feedback, and the students' challenges in completing any assignment along with the student's understandings of the conflicting demands teachers face led to an understanding of how their concerns were more alike than different. The teacher and the students were then able to explore ways to create fewer but more meaningful assignments for both of them.

Thus, although the various interpretive pedagogies are informed by different commitments, they converge in their focus on improving the learning climate, on how teacher and student experience teaching and learning in contemporary health professions schools. Using interpretive pedagogies calls on teachers and students to "put their heads together" to better the learning climate in schools. However, without specific suggestions on how to develop new strategies to bring these pedagogies into the classroom, they will remain difficult to adapt to actual classroom situations (Gore, 1992). The studies in this volume provide actual examples and possibilities for teachers and students to consider.

The interpretive pedagogies advocate student participation in curriculum, instruction, and governance. Attention is given to creating new egalitarian and emancipatory partnerships in which faculty can minimize their power over students and teach in ways that render them simultaneously learners *with* students. The interpretive pedagogies provide ways for teachers to shift from the teacher-as-learner (a familiar role for teachers who often learn from their students) to the learner-as-teacher in which the teacher studies *how* students are learning the content, not just *what* they are learning (Diekelmann, 1991; Diekelmann, 2001; Diekelmann & Ironside, 1998; Stevenson & Beech, 2001; Swenson & Sims, 2000). As a consequence, how a pedagogy influences the learning climate and how students learn becomes a central concern for teachers enacting interpretive pedagogies. Interpretive pedagogies also show teachers how it is possible to intend to be helpful and supportive to students but to behave in ways that have the opposite effect. By shifting the focus from what a teacher might have meant to do to what she or he in fact did, defensiveness can be reduced and efforts made to improve teaching practice.

Currently many faculty in the health professions believe that if they work hard individually to engage students in their classrooms and get good evaluations there is no urgency for reform. Furthermore, many faculty see little need to attend to the communities out of which they practice or the larger learning climate of the school. The relationship between the community teachers create among themselves and the learning climate of the school and how this relationship influences student learning is often devalued, undertheorized, and unexplored. Teachers frequently see little relationship between what is taught (and how it is taught) in the classroom and what students experience in clinical settings other than the simplistic corresponding relationship between the presentation of content in course lectures and its application in clinical settings. Classroom climates (and school climates) are virtually ignored.

This book gathers the interpretive scholarship of researchers exploring new pedagogies for the health professions. Written for students and teachers interested in understanding the contemporary challenges in health professions education and in how research in the interpretive pedagogies can offer new partnerships across healthcare disciplines, it reflects the state of the science of interpretive pedagogies and embraces the latest thinking in, and the utilization of the tenets of, interpretive pedagogies in the health professions in both theoretical and practical ways.

The End of Health Professions Education

Spanos (1993) contends education has reached its end. The end, as used here, is not to be understood as a mere stopping, a lack of continuation, or even a decline or dissolution. Rather, the end of education is the completion of an approach, specifically when all possibilities within an approach have been realized. In this case, subsequent reform becomes merely a matter of inconsequential changes that do not substantively extend or enhance the approach.

While it is impossible to know when (and if) an approach has come to an end (exhausted its possibilities), this book seeks a fresh understanding of "end" to reveal new ways of thinking about reforming health professions education. While many of the studies challenge conventional pedagogy and prophesy an end to outcomes education, it is a different sense of "end" that is ultimately revealed in the interpretive pedagogies. This new understanding of "end" offers alternative ways to think about and create reform. Referring to the end of philosophy, Heidegger (1969/1993), a noted interpretive phenomenologist, comments:

The old meaning of the word "end" means the same as place: "from one end to the other" means: from one place to the other. The end of philosophy is the place, that place in which the whole of philosophy's history is gathered in its most extreme possibility. End as completion means this gathering. (p. 433)

The studies in this book gather new thinking about the nature of reform in the health professions. They share a commitment to explore what it means that conventional pedagogies in health professions education have entered their final stage. The studies ask, "If outcomes education in the health professions has reached its completion, what task is reserved for thinking at the end?" Have we taken outcomes education in the health professions as far as it can go? Are the problems now faced in the classroom and clinical courses such that new pedagogies are needed? Thought of in this way, the end is also a new beginning.

Currently, through the amazing accomplishments of teachers and clinicians in the health sciences, excellent learning experiences prepare students to safely enter the health professions. Often in a very short period of time, with declining resources and increased patient acuity, teachers work tirelessly to prepare students for the demands of future practice. On the other hand, perhaps contemporary health professions education gathers the most extreme possibilities of conventional pedagogies. Perhaps innovations and discoveries such as problem-based learning and instructional technologies (Web-based synchronous and asynchronous courses) are largely returns to an early commitment of conventional pedagogies; specifically learning AS cognitive gain. In conventional pedagogies in the health professions, scientific knowledge is privileged and learning objectives or outcomes shape and frame educational experiences. Evaluation is closely linked with learning objectives, and approaches are sought that are effective and efficient.

This book challenges that approach as a narrow one. Health professions education does not question the commitments conventional pedagogies make to scientific knowledge and a scientific attitude that is tech-nological. This book proposes to be open to how critiquing the assumptions of science are central to exploring the limits of conventional pedagogy even as curricula are challenged to better prepare students in science and scientific approaches to healthcare. Perhaps the greatest danger is that the more teachers become at home in the sciences, the less they question them.

Are the interpretive pedagogies challenges to science and to scien-tific ways of thinking? Yes and no. They are perhaps new ways of think-ing about schooling, learning, and teaching in the health professions that hold open how science is taught and experienced in the curriculum. The question is, "How can teachers prepare for this new thinking (new pedagogies) that thinks the unthought and thinks substantively anew?" The studies in this book illustrate actual situations in which teachers and students co-create or enact new pedagogies. In the data presented, ways to explore new thinking about common problems are described. But there are no new founding frameworks offered to be applied acon-textually, only a kind of preparatory thinking that teachers can bring to their situations as they create site-specific pedagogies. It is not the intent of these collective studies to advocate a universalizing approach. Rather, what should be awakened in the reader is a kind of thinking that is *a readiness* for substantive reform; the recognition of the *contour of this reform*, however, will remain *obscure* and its *coming uncertain*. Heideg-ger (1969/1993) writes: "Thinking must first learn what remains re-served and in store for thinking to get involved in. It prepares its own transformation in this learning" (p. 436).

Interpretive Pedagogies: New Approaches to Health Professions Educa-tion calls educators from all the health professions into converging con-versations in order to create a new future of possibilities for schooling that responds to contemporary challenges. Converging conversations are committed to practical discourses that, describing the wisdom and practical knowledge gained through experiences in schooling, learning, and teaching, can be utilized in reforming health professions education (Diekelmann, 2001; Diekelmann & Diekelmann, forthcoming). Based on past and current experiences, what is in store for us to think about in health professions education? How can this thinking be embraced? Is the call to develop new pedagogies for health professions education a call to thinking anew? This book shows how substantive innovation does not just extend or repackage conventional approaches like lecturing through PowerPoint and Web-based learning activities. The teacher-centeredness of conventional pedagogies is challenged in every study in this book.

Is health professions education at an end? Research indicates (Diekelmann, Allen, & Tanner, 1989; Diekelmann, 2001; Diekelmann & Diekelmann, forthcoming) that significant challenges to conventional pedagogies remain even as "reform" and "innovation" thrive. Perhaps this is because what remains unchallenged in most instructional and curricular reform are the assumptions of conventional pedagogy. Therefore, innovation within this approach does little substantively to address the limitations. Currently, in higher education, new pedagogies (critical, feminist, phenomenological, and postmodern) challenge conventional pedagogies and simultaneously bring research from higher education to bear on the health professions. Critiques of outcomes education are ubiquitous.

Creating a Science of Health Professions Education

There is a dearth of evidence-based health professions education, yet the health sciences disciplines are committed to evidence-based practice (Stevens & Cassidy, 1999). The interpretive studies in this book offer research-based approaches intended to help create a science for health professions education. In Chapter 1, "Converging Conversations from Phenomenological Pedagogies: Toward a Science of Health Professions Education," Karin Dahlberg, Margaretha Ekebergh, and Pamela Ironside describe two research-based pedagogies in nursing, Lifeworld Pedagogy and Narrative Pedagogy, both of which are phenomenological pedagogies. In addition to being research-based, these pedagogies are also discipline-specific.

Specific pedagogies are appearing in the research literature in the health professions (Bligh, Lloyd-Jones, & Smith, 2000; Maudsley & Strivens, 2000; Whipp, Ferguson, Wells, & Iacopino, 2000). Nursing as a discipline is a compelling example of this movement (Dahlberg, Drew, & Nystrom, 2001; Diekelmann, 2001; Diekelmann & Diekelmann, forthcoming). Dahlberg, Ekebergh, and Ironside review the interpretive phenomenological research that generated Lifeworld Pedagogy and Narrative Pedagogy. These studies, undertaken across continents, philosophical traditions, and educational environments, reflect discipline-specific pedagogies and draw attention to thinking about discipline nonspecific pedagogies. Is it the case that one learns medicine in the same way one learns mathematics or geography or botany? Are there theories that apply only to learning a particular discipline? Does one learn nursing the same as one learns medicine or pharmacy?

Embedded in the exegeses of these two discipline-specific pedagogies is a converging conversation that reveals both the dangers (limitations) as well as the benefits (assets). Contained in the interpretations are the contributions of phenomenological pedagogies to the "state of the science" that show how a discipline-specific pedagogy does *not* mean disciplinary nationalism or isolationism but an openness to the question of how these pedagogies advance epistemology and practice in discipline-specific contexts (McPhee & Nohr, 2000). The advantages of these discipline-specific pedagogies are made all the more compelling in light of how universalizing teaching and learning theories cover over and disregard nuanced differences. Rather than comparing and contrasting pedagogies in a battle to select the best, teachers create converging conversations among all pedagogies to extend thinking. Interpretive pedagogies—in holding everything open and problematic, including a postmodern critique of "pedagogies"—foster a respectfulness wherein ideas can be considered and critiqued without the meaningfulness of conventional pedagogies being deconstructed and devalued.

Historical Pathways: Pedagogies Shaped by Disciplinary Practices

In "Mirrors: A Cultural and Historical Interpretation of Nursing's Pedagogies"(Chapter 2), Kathryn Kavanagh provides an historical exegesis of nursing education, yielding important insights into how contemporary healthcare practices influence contemporary health professions education. Historiography, by its very nature, is interpretive. This study provides a model for health professions disciplines to use to explicate the histories of pedagogies within a discipline-specific context. In explicating the path of pedagogies over time, the healthcare professions disciplines can illuminate and open up for critique current assumptions and taken-for granted practices. Important assumptions that are so close at hand they are missed show up in critical historical interpretive studies.

The strength of this volume is that the studies reflect the pluralistic nature of interpretive methodologies. Historical methodologies, critical theory, hermeneutics, feminist, and postmodern discourse analyses, grounded theory, and qualitative description including a multi-methods approach raise important questions about contemporary health professions education. All of the studies offer models for future research as well as outline specific reforms for health professions education.

Teacher and Practitioner Preparation in the Health Professions Education

How clinical practices within a healthcare discipline shape interpretive pedagogies is covered in Chapter 3, "Listening to Learn: Narrative Strategies and Practices in Clinical Education" by Melinda Swenson and Sharon Sims. Their study of the Narrative-Centered Curriculum and narrative strategies and practices in clinical education demonstrates a commitment to not separating practice and teaching. In fact, in the Narrative-Centered Curriculum the central focus is on the dialogues that shape practice, the curriculum-as dialogue. In this study specific narrative instructional strategies using interpretive pedagogies are described in the context of a family nurse practitioner program. The study illuminates how seamlessly wed clinical practice, teaching, and research are as lived.

Students' experiences with interpretive pedagogies and how these experiences shape clinical practice and affect teacher preparation are illustrated in stories of students and teachers. Teacher preparation in the new pedagogies when students have only experienced conventional approaches makes the limitations of "teaching as we were taught," so common in new teachers, even more obvious. The separation of teaching and clinical practice can lead to a devaluing of both. It is only in the web of possibilities created when teaching, research, and practice gather together that new possibilities for each emerge.

Converging Conversations: Pluralistic Methodologies for Health Professions Research

Rose McEldowney, in "Critical Resistance Pathways: Overcoming Oppression in Nursing Education" (Chapter 4), uses feminist discourses and critical theory to expose oppression in nursing education. Critical theory and critical feminist research are central to the interpretive pedagogies in that they challenge and set forth new ways to overcome some of the problems created by conventional pedagogies. McEldowney describes critical resistance pathways with markers that reveal oppression in nursing education. The critical resistance pathways are self-critical and reveal the ever-present oppression and silencing even within efforts to reform. The converging conversations created by critical feminist interpretive pedagogies demonstrate that one can study oneself in self-reflexive scholarship. How "the personal is political" is explicated in the interpretations of narratives.

Creating a Science for Health Professions Education

In the science-based health professions, medical science and nursing science are commonplace phrases. Yet there is no science of medical education or science of nursing education. It is time to begin creating a research base for health professions education. Toward that end, interpretive studies extend, reaffirm, and challenge scientific studies while contributing to a research base. While this book predominantly gathers interpretive studies aimed at developing a science for health education, in studies such as Chapter 5, "Teaching as Nourishment for Complex Thought: Approaches for Classroom and Practice Built on Postformal Theory and the Creation of Community," Jan Sinnott shows how multimethod research adds important dimensions to both scientific and interpretive studies. Postformal Theory includes both interpretive and scientific approaches and thus makes contributions to evidence-based teaching and learning as well as offers interpretations of meanings and significances in schooling experiences. In this way, Sinnott describes how scientific theories can be used in ways that support and encourage interpretive pedagogies.

Research in the interpretive pedagogies that is pluralistic and multimethod holds open revisioning new partnerships and engendering communities of health professions students, teachers, and practitioners. Deconstruction and critique are vital to reforming health professions education but so is identifying the strengths of conventional pedagogies. Research in the interpretive pedagogies that reveals the similarities and common practices of schooling, learning, and teaching in the health professions illuminates the converging rather than the contesting conversations. Both conversations are needed if a science in health professions education is to be elucidated. Contesting conversations about pedagogies critique, keep open, and deconstruct practices of power and oppression. Converging conversations are self-reflective in that they recover the embodied or lived experiences of schooling, learning, and teaching. These unending conversations are historically situated, bringing all pedagogies to bear through dialogue and debate in an effort to create a neoteric health professions education.

References

American Association of Colleges of Nursing. (1995). *The essentials of master's education for advanced practice nursing.* Washington, DC: American Association of Colleges of Nursing.

Andrews, C. A., Ironside, P. M., Nosek, C., Sims, S. L., Swenson, M. M., Yeomans, C., et al. (2001). Enacting narrative pedagogy: The lived experiences of students and teachers. *Nursing and Health Care Perspectives, 22*(5), 252–259.

Apple, M. W. (2001). *Educating the "right way": Markets, standards, God, and inequality.* New York: RoutledgeFalmer.

Armstrong, E. G., & Koffman, R. G. (2000). Enhancing nutrition education through faculty development: From workshops to Web sites. *American Journal of Clinical Nutrition, 72*(3 Suppl), S877–S881.

Atwell-Vasey, W. (1998). *Nourishing words: Bridging private reading and public teaching.* Albany: State University of New York Press.

Barr, R., & Tagg, J. (1995). From learning to teaching: A new paradigm for undergraduate education. *Change, 27,* 13–25.

Benner, P., Hooper-Kyriakidis, P., & Stannard, D. (1999). *Clinical wisdom and interventions in critical care: A thinking-in-action approach.* Philadelphia: W. B. Saunders.

Berger, C. S., & Ai, A. (2000). Managed care and its implications for social work curricula reform: Clinical practice and field instruction. *Social Work Health Care, 31*(3), 83–106.

Bligh, J., Lloyd-Jones, G., & Smith, G. (2000). Early effects of a new problem-based clinically oriented curriculum on students' perceptions of teaching. *Medical Education, 34*(6), 487–489.

Boyer Commission on Educating Undergraduates. (2000). *Reinventing undergraduate education: A blueprint for America's research universities.* New York: Boyer Commission on Educating Undergraduates.

Bromley, H., & Apple, M. E. (Eds.). (1998). *Education/Technology/Power: Educational computing as a social practice.* Albany: State University of New York Press

Carlson, D., & Apple, M. W. (Eds.). (1998). *Power/knowledge/pedagogy: The meaning of democratic education in unsettling times.* Boulder, CO: Westview Press.

Castells, M., Flecha, R., Freire, P., Giroux, H., Macedo, D., & Willis, P. (1999). *Critical education in the new information age.* Lanham, MD: Rowman & Littlefield Publishers.

Choudry, U. K. (1992). New nurse faculty: Core competencies in role development. *Journal of Nursing Education, 31*, 26–30.

Cohee, G. E., Daumer, E., Kemp, T., Krebs, P., Lafky, S. A., & Runzo, S. (Eds.). (1998). *The feminist teachers anthology: Pedagogies and classroom strategies.* New York: Teachers College Press.

Creager, A., Lunbeck, E., & Schiebinger, L. (Eds.). (2001). Feminism in twentieth century science, technology, and medicine. Chicago: University of Chicago Press.

Dahlberg, K., Drew, N., & Nystrom, M. (2001). *Reflective lifeworld research.* Lund: Studentlitteratur.

DeSevo, M. R. (1995). Part-time nursing faculty: Suggestions for change. *Journal of Nursing Education, 34*(7), 294–296.

DeYoung, S., & Bliss, J. B. (1995). Nursing faculty: An endangered species? *Journal of Professional Nursing, 11*(2), 84–88.

Diekelmann, N. (1991). The emancipatory power of the narrative. In *Curriculum revolution: Community building and activism.* New York: National League for Nursing Press.

Diekelmann, N. (2001). Narrative pedagogy: Heideggerian hermeneutical analyses of the lived experiences of students, teachers, and clinicians. *Advances in Nursing Science, 23*(3), 53–71.

Diekelmann, N. (2002) "Pitching a lecture" and "reading the faces of students": Learning lecturing and the embodied practices of teaching. *Journal of Nursing Education, 41*(3), 97–99.

Diekelmann, N., Allen, D., & Tanner, C. (1989). The National League for Nursing criteria for appraisal of baccalaureate programs: A critical hermeneutic analysis. In L. Moody & M. Shannon (Eds.), *NLN Nursing Research Monograph Series.* New York: National League for Nursing Press. (Refereed.)

Diekelmann, N., & Diekelmann, J. (forthcoming). *Schooling learning teaching: Toward a Narrative Pedagogy.* Madison: University of Wisconsin Press.

Diekelmann, N., & Ironside, P. M. (1998). Preserving writing in doctoral education: Exploring the concernful practices of schooling learning teaching. *Journal of Advanced Nursing, 28*(6), 1347–1355.

Donovan, J. (2001). *Feminist theory.* New York: Continuum.

Eitel, F., Kanz, K. G., Hortig, E., & Tesche, A. (2000). Do we face a fourth paradigm shift in medicine—algorithms in education? *Journal of Evaluation of Clinical Practices, 6*(3), 321–333.

Fox, R. C. (1999). Time to heal medical education? *Academic Medicine, 74*(10), 1072–1075.

Giroux, H. (1997). Where have all the public intellectuals gone? Racial politics, pedagogy, and disposable youth. *Journal of Composition Theory, 17*, 191–205.

Gore, J. (1992). *The struggle for pedagogies: Critical and feminist discourses as regimes of truth.* New York: Routledge.

Haroutunian-Gordon, S. (1998). A study of reflective thinking: Patterns in interpretive discussion. *Educational Theory, 48*, 33–58.

Hartrick, G. (2000). Developing health-promoting practice with families: One pedagogical experience. *Journal of Advanced Nursing, 31*(1), 27–34.

Heidegger, M. (1969/1993). The end of philosophy and the task of thinking (Rev. ed.). In D. Krell (Ed. & Trans.), *Basic writings* (pp. 433, 436). San Francisco: Harper.

Hillocks, G. (1999). *Ways of thinking, ways of teaching.* New York: Teacher's College Press.

hooks, b. (2000). *Where we stand: Class matters.* New York: Routledge.

Iglehart, J. (2000). Forum on the future of academic medicine: final session—implications of the information revolution for academic medicine. *Academic Medicine,* 75(3), 245–251.

Ironside, P. M. (1997). *Preserving reading, writing, thinking, and dialogue: Rethinking doctoral education in nursing.* Unpublished doctoral dissertation, University of Wisconsin–Madison.

Ironside, P. M. (2001). Creating a research base for nursing education: An interpretive review of conventional, critical, feminist, postmodern, and phenomenologic pedagogies. *Advances in Nursing Science, 23*(3), 72–87.

Jones, A., McArdle, P. J., & O'Neill, P. A. (2002). Perceptions of how well graduates are prepared for the role of pre-registration house officer: A comparison of outcomes from a traditional and an integrated PBL curriculum. *Medical Education, 36*(1), 16–25.

Kassebaum, D. G., & Cutler, E. R. (1998). On the culture of student abuse in medical school. *Academic Medicine, 73*(11), 1149–1158.

Kerdeman, D. (1998). Hermeneutics and education: Understanding, control, and agency. *Educational Theory, 48*(2), 241–266.

Kincheloe, J. L., & Steinberg, S. R. (Eds.). (1998). *Unauthorized methods: Strategies for critical teaching.* New York: Routledge.

Lesky, L., & Yonke, A. (2001). The Interdisciplinary Generalist Curriculum Project at the University of Illinois at Chicago College of Medicine. *Academic Medicine, 76*(4 Suppl), S117–S120.

Maudsley, G., & Strivens, J. (2000). Promoting professional knowledge, experiential learning, and critical thinking for medical students. *Medical Education, 34*(7), 535–544.

Mayberry, M., & Rose, E. C. (Eds.). (1999). *Meeting the challenge: Innovative feminist pedagogies in action.* New York: Routledge.

McEwan, H., & Egan, K. (Eds.). (1995). *Narrative in teaching, learning, and research.* New York: Teacher's College Press.

McPhee, W., & Nohr, C. (2000). Globalization and the cultural impact on distance education. *International Journal of Medical Information, 58–59,* 291–295.

Nehls, N. (1995). Narrative pedagogy: Rethinking nursing education. *Journal of Nursing Education, 34*(5), 204–210.

Neistadt, M. E. (1999). Educational interpretation of "cooperative learning as an approach to pedagogy." *American Journal of Occupational Therapists, 53*(1), 41–43.

Noddings, N. (2002). *Educating moral people: A caring alternative to character education.* New York: Teachers College Press.

Norton, S. F., & Spross, J. A. (1994). From advanced practice to academia: Developmental tasks and strategies for role socialization. *Journal of Nursing Education, 33*(8), 373–375.

Opdycke, S. (1999). *No one was turned away.* New York: Oxford University Press.

Plater, W. (1995). Future work: Faculty time in the 21st century. *Change, 27*(3), 23–33.

Post, D. (1997). *Nurse Educators 1997: Findings from the RN and LPN Faculty Census.* Boston: John Bartlett.

Post, D., & Louden, D. (1997). *Nursing Data Review: 1997.* New York: National League for Nursing Press.

Princeton, J. C. (1992). The teacher crisis in nursing education—revisited. *Nurse Educator, 17*(5), 34–37.

Ryan, M., & Irvine, P. (1994). Nursing professorate in America: Projected retirements and replacements. *Journal of Nursing Education, 33*(2), 67–73.

Shatzer, J. H. (1998). Instructional methods. *Academic Medicine, 73*(9 Suppl), S38–S45.

Sheehe, J. B., & Schoener, L. (1994). Risk and reality for nurse educators. *Holistic Nursing Practice, 8*(2), 53–58.

Shor, I. (1986). Equality is excellence: Transforming teacher education and the learning process. *Harvard Educational Review, 56,* 406–426.

Smith, A., & Webster, F. E. (Eds.). (1997). *The postmodern university? Contested visions of higher education in society.* Buckingham, UK: Open University Press.

Spanos, W. V. (1993). *The end of education: Toward post-humanism.* Minneapolis: University of Minnesota Press.

Stevens, K. R., & Cassidy, V. R. (1999). *Evidenced-based teaching: Current research in nursing education.* New York: National League for Nursing Press.

Stevenson, C., & Beech, I. (2001). Paradigms lost, paradigms regained: Defending nursing against a single reading of postmodernism. *Nursing Philosophy, 2,* 143–150.

Swenson, M. M., & Sims, S. L. (2000). Toward a narrative-centered curriculum for nurse practitioners. *Journal of Nursing Education, 39*(3), 109–115.

van Manen, M. (1991). Reflectivity and the pedagogical moment: The normativity of pedagogical thinking and acting. *Journal of Curriculum Studies, 23*(6), 507–536.

Whipp, J. L., Ferguson, D. J., Wells, L. M., & Iacopino, A. M. (2000). Rethinking knowledge and pedagogy in dental education. *Journal of Dental Education, 64*(12), 860–866.

Young, P. K. (1999). *Joining the academic community: The lived experiences of new teachers.* Unpublished doctoral dissertation, University of Wisconsin–Madison.

1

Converging Conversations from Phenomenological Pedagogies

Toward a Science of Health Professions Education

Karin Dahlberg, Margaretha Ekebergh, and Pamela M. Ironside

The discipline of nursing, like all health sciences, is firmly committed to developing a science for practice. Serious scholarship in nursing continues to expand the body of knowledge (evidence) upon which practicing nurses can draw to insure their practice is research-based. But, does this commitment extend to nursing education? Should there be a science of health professions education? Should teaching in the health science disciplines be research-based? Examining these questions is imperative given the challenges facing schools of nursing worldwide, including (a) a nursing shortage and the concomitant demands to increase student enrollments, (b) increasing diversity among matriculated students, (c) constant change in healthcare delivery systems, (d) a critical teacher shortage, and (e) the common imperative for nurses and nurse teachers to do more with fewer resources. Virtually every school of nursing is attempting to meet these challenges by implementing significant curricular and/or instructional reform. Is this reform evidence-based? Is reform in nursing education guided by the best available research and theories developed in both higher and nursing education? Are implemented reform efforts being comprehensively examined to determine their efficacy and meaningfulness in meeting the contemporary

22

challenges of teaching nursing practice? Without a strong disciplinary commitment to developing a science of nursing education, those implementing reform will be doing so based on trial and error or anecdotal evidence rather than on evidence that is research-based, systematic, and longitudinal. Yet, the very presence of ongoing reform holds open the possibility of a science of nursing education.

This study presents an exegesis of two ongoing research programs—one from the United States and one from Scandinavia—that contribute to and extend the science of nursing education. Diekelmann (1995, 2001) has developed Narrative Pedagogy, a research-based interpretive phenomenological approach to schooling, learning, and teaching based in continental philosophy that emerged out of her hermeneutical analysis of the lived experiences of teachers, students, and clinicians as recorded in interviews. Ekebergh (2001) has developed Lifeworld Pedagogy, a research-based educational model within the framework of phenomenology and European caring theory (Eriksson, 1987, 1990, 1993; Eriksson & Lindström, 2000). By exploring the philosophical and epistemological commitments of these new pedagogies, the authors elucidate the commonalities and differences between these approaches and describe how discovering and enacting new discipline-specific pedagogies affords the possibility of contributing to the science of education for the health professions.

Method

This study explores the use of phenomenological philosophy as described by Husserl, Heidegger, Merleau-Ponty, and Gadamer transformed into a phenomenological scientific research approach and as a way of explicating the phenomena of teaching and learning. With this approach we analyzed enactments of Lifeworld Pedagogy in Scandinavia and Narrative Pedagogy in the United States, which were described in written texts revealing the converging conversations that also illuminated the philosophical underpinnings and empirical backgrounds of these pedagogies. The descriptions were augmented by the inclusion of exemplars from the databases created during the conduct of these international studies.

During the analysis of Lifeworld Pedagogy and Narrative Pedagogy new understandings became apparent as we began reading across the texts from both studies. A number of common themes emerged, which we synthesized into a single text. The new readings of common themes led us to further explore and describe the similarities and differences in the two phenomenological pedagogies. For instance, both Lifeworld Pedagogy and Narrative Pedagogy emphasize the importance of reflection in the context of learning in nursing, yet how reflection is enacted within each pedagogical approach differs. In Lifeworld Pedagogy, reflection is an "act of embodied consciousness"; in Narrative Pedagogy, reflection is a community practice of thinking evoked through storytelling (narrative interpretations). Similarly, differing international viewpoints enriched our understanding as we explicated common teaching and learning practices on two continents into a new written text. The conversation between Swedish and English further served the interpretive process as we had to create a common language to describe our thinking in ways that extended or affirmed particular national usage.

Dialogue among us as co-authors served to fill out and expand on the new interpretations of common themes and to challenge or critique them—often leading us back to rethink our analysis of the text, our experiences enacting these new pedagogies, and the philosophical underpinnings giving rise to this scholarship. The ongoing dialogue also served to affirm the importance of the international converging conversations about the new discipline-specific phenomenological pedagogies wherein teacher-scholars reflect on the commitments and assumptions embedded in approaches to teaching and how these pedagogies are enacted in learning encounters. Further, these converging conversations encouraged the further development of these discipline-specific pedagogies and contributed to a science of education for the health professions.

Narrative Pedagogy

Since 1988 Diekelmann has been conducting research in nursing education by using Heideggerian hermeneutics to explicate the lived experiences of teachers, students, and clinicians. Throughout this time, data have been collected via audiotaped, nonstructured interviews with more than 250 teachers and students representing all levels of nursing education and with more than 100 clinicians from a wide variety of practice specialties. Participants were asked to describe memorable experiences in the context of nursing education. The audiotaped interviews were transcribed verbatim by an experienced transcriptionist for analysis. These transcribed accounts have constituted the data for this longitudinal program of research.

Diekelmann has consistently utilized a research team to bring multiple perspectives to bear on the analysis. While membership of the research team has varied over the past thirteen years, the composition of the team has remained consistent: teachers and students, other interpretive researchers, and a continuing education specialist. Analyzing data using Heideggerian hermeneutical phenomenology, the research team has uncovered the common experiences and shared meanings of nursing education as described by teachers, students, and clinicians. The hermeneutic method for analyzing texts is briefly described below, although the reader is referred to other texts that describe this methodology in detail (Benner, Tanner, & Chesla, 1996; Diekelmann, Allen, & Tanner, 1989; Diekelmann & Ironside, 1998a; Grondin, 1990; MacLeod, 1996).

The hermeneutic analysis begins with team members reading each interview text to gain an overall understanding of the participant's experience and to identify common themes. Themes describe recurrent categories or ideas that reflect the shared experiences and practices embedded within the text (Diekelmann & Ironside, 1998a). During research-team meetings, team members read the themes they identified and their interpretation of these themes aloud. Each team member supports her or his interpretation of identified themes with excerpts from the interview text. As subsequent texts are analyzed, team members discuss the commonalities and differences emerging in the interpretations. Team members clarify vague, unclear, or conflicting meanings that surface during the analysis by referring back to the interview text or by reinterviewing the participants.

As they continued their analysis of the interview texts, team members investigated recurrent themes—those themes that were identified across multiple texts—more fully, challenging and elaborating on the interpretations using critical, feminist, and postmodern literature; the philosophical texts of Heidegger, Gadamer, and Merleau Ponty; and the extant literature from nursing and higher education. The point of bringing this variety of texts to bear on emerging themes was not to seek one correct interpretation but to add richness and complexity to the interpretation by exploring nuances and qualitative distinctions present across multiple texts (Diekelmann & Ironside, 1998a) and to insure the interpretations were situated within current knowledge and practice.

During the interpretive analysis of the study data the Concernful Practices of Schooling, Learning, and Teaching emerged as patterns (Table 1). (A pattern is the highest level of hermeneutic analysis; it is constitutive in that it expresses the relationship between the themes, and it is present in all interview texts [Diekelmann & Ironside, 1998a].) As patterns, the Concernful Practices describe the common experiences and shared meanings of teachers, students, and clinicians in nursing education. *Concernful*, here, is used in the Heideggerian sense of describing what matters, what is of concern, or what calls for thought. Thus, the Concernful Practices provide teachers, students, and clinicians with a new language for describing what matters about schooling, learning, and teaching, one that fosters the ongoing exploration of the meanings and significances of their educational experiences. The Concernful Practices continue to be explicated (Diekelmann & Diekelmann, 2001) and enacted in a variety of settings (Andrews et al, 2001; Diekelmann, 2001; Diekelmann & Ironside, 1998b; Ironside, 1997; Kavanagh 1998; Swenson & Sims, 2000; Young, 1998).

During the course of this longitudinal study, Diekelmann began to publicly share stories that illuminated particular Concernful Practices in "all school" meetings (Voices Day) at seven international schools of nursing as a way to elicit converging conversations among students, teachers, and clinicians. In so doing, Diekelmann discovered a new pedagogy she called Narrative Pedagogy. Voices Day participants reported

Table 1 The Concernful Practices of Schooling, Learning, and Teaching

Gathering: Bringing in and calling forth

Creating Places: Keeping open a future of possibilities

Assembling: Constructing and cultivating

Staying: Knowing and connecting

Caring: Engendering community

Interpreting: Unlearning and becoming

Presencing: Attending and being open

Preserving: Reading, writing, thinking, and dialogue

Questioning: Meaning and making visible

Source: N. Diekelmann, 2001

that when they gathered to collectively share and interpret their experiences their community life substantively changed and their understanding of how others experienced nursing education was enhanced. This understanding fostered new partnerships between and among teachers, students, and clinicians that reformed and extended current educational practices (Diekelmann, 2001; Diekelmann & Diekelmann, 2000; Ironside, 1999, 2001). Consequently, Voices Day participants contributed to the discovery of Narrative Pedagogy and to the rigor of Diekelmann's research by affirming the significance of the Concernful Practices and by supporting, extending, clarifying, and challenging her interpretations in the context of contemporary nursing education.

Understood in this way, Narrative Pedagogy is a research-based, interpretive phenomenological approach to schooling, learning, and teaching that was developed *from* nursing research *for* nursing education (Andrews et al., 2001; Ironside, 2001). Narrative Pedagogy arises out of conducting a regional ontology of schooling, learning, and teaching in the context of nursing education. In addition to Narrative Pedagogy being an approach to schooling, learning, and teaching, it is a way of thinking and a community practice that arises when teachers and students gather to share and interpret stories from their lived experiences in nursing education. Thus, interpreting narratives creates a dialogue among teachers, students, and clinicians that is reflective, reflexive, and focused on common practices. This dialogue illuminates for the participants times of "getting through," times of making a difference in each other's lives, and times of breakdown when "nothing went right." As teachers, students, and clinicians consider these times of connecting and times of breakdown, they enhance their understanding of each other's experiences within the school of nursing. This understanding, in the Heideggerian sense, is not static, final, and conclusive but dynamic and fluid as the shared practices of learning are persistently held open and problematic. This openness creates a future of new possibilities for nursing education.

It is important to note, however, that Narrative Pedagogy arises out of and co-occurs with conventional pedagogies (outcomes or competency-based education) as well as with critical, feminist, phenomenological, and postmodern pedagogies (Diekelmann, 2001; Ironside, 2001). Similarly, because Narrative Pedagogy occurs when teachers, students, and clinicians collectively share and interpret their experiences of teaching and learning, it is always site-specific and situated. It is unique in each situation in which it occurs and therefore defies precise definition, articulation, or evaluation. However the process of *how* Narrative Pedagogy is enacted can be generalized (Diekelmann & Diekelmann, 2002; Diekelmann, 2001). Narrative Pedagogy is not a strategy to be implemented but rather a way to create an environment within nursing education that invites teachers, students, and clinicians into converging conversations. Narrative Pedagogy also gathers all pedagogies into converging conversations when teachers, students, and clinicians interpret their experiences together and remain open to the possibility for anything to emerge. Thus, it is out of individual and community reflective scholarship that Narrative Pedagogy arises.

Lifeworld Pedagogy

The Scandinavian study (Ekebergh, 2001) was conducted at three schools of nursing in Sweden and Finland. The research was carried out using a phenomenological approach (Giorgi, 1997; Dahlberg et al., 2001). Data were collected in the form of written accounts and interviews with students both in the nursing program, which confers a baccalaureate degree in caring science, and in the master's (MA) program of caring science. The phenomenon under study was the process of acquiring caring-science knowledge or, more precisely, the integration of theoretical knowledge with knowledge within healthcare practice. The epistemological concerns that anchor nursing education were explicated in this study with the goal of illuminating the common "gap" between caring-science theory and praxis. The phenomenological approach found expression in terms of openness and pliability during this research in relation to the phenomenon and the informants. The interviews began in the lifeworld of the students, and the interview questions asked by the researcher directed the awareness of the student to the area under investigation and deepened the lifeworld descriptions offered by the students. Such openness required the researcher to be aware of how her pre-understanding (Dahlberg et al., 2001) might influence the study. Thus, during the entire study the researcher's aim was to keep this pre-understanding in check or to "bridle" it to the extent possible (Dahlberg et al., 2001).

In accordance with the approach, the research was further characterized by the search for essences, or that which makes the phenomenon the phenomenon (Dahlberg et al., 2001). The understanding of a phenomenon in terms of its essence demands from the researcher an openness that allows the phenomenon to show itself and its characteristics. This means, for example, that the researcher needs to remain sensitive to the implicit but emerging structure of meanings and avoid interpretation and speculation. Consequently, the researcher strives to stay as close to the meaning of the data as possible throughout the study.

The results of this research described the general structure of the phenomenon and explicated how the students' process of learning was characterized by solitariness. Solitariness ensued when the students, as bearers of theoretical knowledge, could not share and work at applying this theoretical knowledge in practice situations with teachers or other caregivers. The students' need for reflection and their desire to understand caring-science knowledge in practice was often disregarded by teachers and caregivers who emphasized student performance. At the master's level, students had the opportunity to enhance their caring-science knowledge within the framework of their educational program, but even they experienced solitariness in caring practice, and little ground for extending caring-science knowledge. However, master's students also reported that the theoretical knowledge of caring enriched their lives in ways that contributed to their personal development and well-being. This was seldom the case for the baccalaureate students, and these students, therefore, suffered greatly from solitariness in their learning.

The students' learning was markedly colored by their personal life experiences and there was an explicit need for them to link caring-science knowledge to these experiences. Not all students succeeded in this, since it requires both a certain degree of personal maturity and insight from the student. It also presupposes that caring-science knowledge is provided in a form that can affect a student's life. Students can develop the maturity that is needed for caring science to be integrated into their lives through reflection on existential problems and on the substance and meaning of life. Caring-science knowledge can, in turn, give an impetus to such reflection, which in favorable circumstances, can support a student's maturation. Caring-science knowledge, however, must be vital and robust in order to take root and grow in the student's world of experience, something that acontextual caring theories cannot achieve. Thus, a balance must be realized between learner and knowledge as a precondition for caring-science knowledge to be implemented in the student's world of experience.

Particularly unfortunate conditions for learning occur when "an immature student" encounters "immature caring-science knowledge" within an "immature pedagogy." The solitariness in learning and the students' frequent difficulty applying theoretical caring knowledge to clinical care exacerbate the problem. A central prerequisite for the integration of caring science into the student's world of experience is personal guidance by a teacher who is well versed in caring science and who can support students as they become conscious of and articulate their lifeworld experience. It is a matter of teachers rendering self-reflection possible for students within their learning encounters before the students are brought face-to-face with caring-science knowledge.

Caring-science knowledge, however, is not always implemented in practice, which has consequences for student learning. Caring science is not made sufficiently lifelike in the didactic relations between students and their clinical teachers. This shortcoming appears clearly in conventional teaching and model learning, which hampers the integrative process of caring-science praxis and its fusion with the student's world of experience. Since knowledge of caring theory is lacking in practical caring contexts, the process of learning caring begins in "common sense" and proceeds through a natural caring stance. Consequently, conscious reflection is all too often dispensed with by teachers, as teachers emphasize student conduct that is unreflective and imitative. The focus of imitative approaches (also called model learning) on "doing" implies that students will only be affirmed in what they concretely perform. Affirmation of a conscious development of caring-science knowledge will not occur in such situations.

The findings of this empirical research, informed by the pairing of a caring-science perspective with an epistemological anchorage in phenomenology, led to the development of a didactic structure that includes three principles intended to encourage the learning and teaching of caring-science knowledge:

1. *Didactics should be rooted in caring-science substance.* That is, caring-science didactics are substance-oriented. The didactics of caring science presents the ethos of caring, which is the core of the learning both with regard to the substance of knowledge and the perspective taken. A consequence

of this principle is that caring-science didactics are never to be understood as mere techniques.

2. *Didactics should recognize the possibility of reflection integrating caring-science knowledge of theory and practice into the world of experience.* In order for the caring-science substance to influence the students' learning, a certain didactic reflection is required that affirms their lifeworld. It is then a question of an experienced, personified reflection, which involves the students and their individual lives.

3. *Didactics should form a relation that makes a learning communion possible.* In order to create a meaningful learning experience, students need the support of a teacher. In a learning relationship caring knowledge can be made vivid, which creates preconditions for it to influence the student and to be integrated into the student's world of experience.

Phenomenology and Pedagogies

The commitment to phenomenology is central to Narrative and Lifeworld Pedagogies emerging from studies in the United States and Scandinavia. Phenomenological pedagogies, which turn on openness, reflectivity, and community practices (or a learning communion between and among teachers and students), are enacted when teachers and students strive to understand how education is experienced (Ironside, 2001). Teachers enacting Narrative Pedagogy and Lifeworld Pedagogy attend to the meanings and significances embedded in the students' experiences of learning nursing. The strength of phenomenological pedagogies lies not in theorizing, generating knowledge, or critiquing other approaches to teaching and learning, but in understanding and exploring what a teacher does and is in relation to students as they learn caring science and nursing. This is not to suggest that such pedagogies do not, in fact, contribute to extending disciplinary epistemologies but rather that such contributions are derivative. In other words, extending epistemologies in health professions education begins by understanding the educational encounter.

Philosophically grounded in phenomenology, as expressed by Husserl and Merleau-Ponty, Lifeworld Pedagogy emphasizes openness to that which shows itself in the context of learning and specifically addresses nursing epistemologies in which traditional views of epistemologies as knowledge systems are replaced by a focus on lived experiences or encounters. As such, Lifeworld Pedagogy begins in an encounter between the learner and the teacher and between learners, teachers, and the "thing" that is the focus of learning and teaching.

Philosophically grounded in Heideggerian (interpretive) phenomenology, Narrative Pedagogy emphasizes understanding the common experiences and shared meanings of schooling, learning, and teaching. Understanding, according to Heidegger, is "the power to grasp one's own possibilities for being within the context of the lifeworld in which one exists" (Palmer, 1969, p. 131). Understanding, then, is always already contextual and is directed toward possibilities. Thus, Narrative Pedagogy gathers teachers, students, and clinicians to collectively share and interpret their common experiences in nursing education in ways that foster new understandings and a future of new possibilities for nursing education.

The science of caring and how it is taught and experienced is the nexus of Lifeworld Pedagogy and Narrative Pedagogy. In both pedagogies, narratives are central and the explication (interpreting) of narratives, both as an individual and community experience, is a process that enacts these pedagogies. In Lifeworld Pedagogy, narratives are considered to be lifeworld narratives—stories, accounts, or other illustrations of lived learning experiences. Lifeworld narratives can be written or oral. They can be in the form of diary notes or can be elicited by questions such as, "tell me a narrative that describes your lived experience of learning." Narratives can be elicited by descriptions of critical events—those strong, often pivotal, situations that are vividly remembered in detail over a long period of time. A good description of a critical event is often more illuminating than a general description of a phenomenon. Narratives can also be elicited through the practice of educational drama (Lepp, Ekebergh, & Dahlberg, 2001). For example, role playing may support the expression of an ambiguous lived learning experience.

Within Narrative Pedagogy, narratives refer to descriptions of lived experiences. These narratives are stories, shared publicly by teachers, students, and clinicians, that are memorable to the one offering the story for their ability to illuminate what matters or what is meaningful in the context of schooling, learning, and teaching. As the story is shared, teachers, students, and clinicians gather to interpret the narrative and in so doing uncover new understandings. In Narrative Pedagogy then, the emphasis is not merely on sharing (or hearing) a particular story but on collectively interpreting the common meanings and significances of the story. Throughout the presentation of this chapter, narratives collected in the context of both Narrative Pedagogy and Lifeworld Pedagogy studies will be provided.

Phenomenological Pedagogies—A General Structure

Openness

Phenomenology is made up of two basic components. The first component is the phenomenological turn to "the thing" being studied, the phenomenon. The second component is the demand for openness or sensitivity to "the things" (Bengtsson, 1998; Dahlberg et al., 2001). Openness is thus the general principle that guides a phenomenology of learning and teaching. In such an approach to learning and teaching, "going to the things themselves" involves turning to the experience of learning and teaching with the aim of gaining an understanding of learners' lifeworlds through their narratives. Instead of teaching scientific theory, common sense, or any pregiven perspectives, teachers using a phenomenological pedagogy try to do justice to and to be open and sensitive to the phenomenon of learning and to the learner.

In the context of pedagogy, openness is the expression of a way of being. It is an attitude or posture that stands in direct contrast to dogmatism. Openness is the mark of receptivity, flexibility and sensitivity, and a true willingness to listen to, and understand the lifeworld of, the learners. It involves respect for and humility toward the phenomenon and the learner.

Heidegger (1927/1962) describes such an open position as a desire to see or to understand the phenomenon. In phenomenological pedagogy, openness is being ready or poised for the possibility of anything showing up. This openness (desire to understand) could also be regarded as a curiosity in relation to and engagement with the world of the learner. For teachers, openness consequently means having the capacity to listen and to be surprised by and sensitive to the unpredictable and unexpected. As a result of the teacher's open stance, the events and objects of the learner's experience may disclose themselves as being different from what they were earlier assumed to be.

In both Lifeworld Pedagogy and Narrative Pedagogy, openness means that teachers and students make themselves receptive and sensitive to the phenomenon of interest as it presents itself (Husserl, 1936/ 1970; Heidegger, 1927/1962; Merleau-Ponty, 1945/1995; Gadamer, 1960/1995). Such an attitude of openness is not easily accomplished because of our common tendency to see events or objects as things that already have meaning, as things we already understand. It is a well-known problem that we do not always see what is there or that we can often be lured into seeing something that does not exist because we assume too quickly that we understand the phenomenon (Dahlberg et al., 2001; Dahlberg & Dahlberg, 2002). Therefore, we must always maintain a reasonable doubt, a persistent tentativeness about how we understand the phenomenon. As Heidegger (1927/1962) contends, there is always the possibility that something will show itself as something that it actually is not. So too, educational situations are marked by their historical, political, and sociocultural context, and teachers as well as students often make assumptions about the learning situation, acting in unreflective ways, which Diekelmann describes as "teaching as we were taught" (personal communication, April 15, 2002). The danger of "teaching as we were taught" is that the assumptions made by teachers and students, the hegemonic influence of institutionalized education, and the historical trajectory of the discipline remain invisible and unchallenged.

To be open refers to the receptivity of the teacher and consequently her or his willingness and ability to engage with the learner, thereby establishing trust between and among teachers and students that allows for the possibility of disclosure. In Narrative Pedagogy, this openness and ability to engage with the learner is reflected in the Concernful Practice of *Presencing: Attending and Being Open*. Instead of controlling the teaching situation, the teacher is open to and prepared to be captivated by student efforts to learn. Such an approach calls for teachers and students to be involved in and present to the learning encounter. This requires teachers to be ready for anything to occur.

In the Scandinavian study, several anecdotes from students demonstrate the value of teachers being open to and connecting with students. This connecting often occurred when teachers decentered themselves and focused on students' learning style. Students frequently recalled experiences in which their desire to be recognized by teachers as individuals was affirmed and supported as they developed their knowledge of nursing practice.

One student described the ideal teacher as one who is:

very attentive to what each student has done before, what kind of background they have. What have they experienced during their life. It is very important.

In an open dialogue with the teacher, a student can share her or his experiences, which gives the teacher some insight into the understanding of the student.

I try to tell what I have done before and what I am not able to handle when I enter a place for my clinical studies, and what I would like to learn and practice. Then she will have a picture of me.

When teachers know students as individuals, they can better support each student when problems appear in the process of learning. Knowing students as individuals also contributes to the student's sense of self-confidence and self-esteem, particularly when a failure is immanent.

Diekelmann's Concernful Practice *Staying: Knowing and Connecting* shows how teachers and students stay in situations with one another by attempting to find connections. Teachers commonly described how they tried to learn about the students' background and past experiences and likewise, students reported how they tried to "get to know" their teachers by finding out "who [the teacher] is as a person." In the context of Narrative Pedagogy, however, the Concernful Practices are neither negative nor positive in themselves. Rather it is how the Concernful Practices are enacted in particular situations that lead them to be experienced as positive or negative. For example, teachers may connect with students by ignoring their backgrounds and previous experiences. In this case, the teacher's approach to knowing the students is a negative one in which the students may feel devalued and isolated. In Narrative Pedagogy, not connecting is considered a kind of connecting. The Concernful Practices describe the common experiences of schooling, learning, and teaching, but it is only in the interpretation of these stories that the meanings and significances become apparent. Stories are always contextual, and what matters about the Concernful Practices is how they are experienced in particular situations.

In the U.S. study, many students recalled how teachers worked diligently to help them learn. Maria, a graduate student, described how, in her struggle to understand course content, a teacher guided her search for understanding.

I'm sitting there crying because here everybody is talking about [nursing theo-rists] and I had no idea who these people were. I had not even a clue who these people were and I went, "I really have to do some background work here." I went up to the instructor with tears in my eyes and I said, "I have no concept of what you are saying, I don't even have a clue." She gave me a stack of books. She gave me about five books and she said, "Well, why don't you read these . . . before you come back next week." And I said "all right." And I went back to her a week later and I said, "I still don't understand." So she gave me St. Thomas Aquinas to read. And I sat there and I really tried. I really tried to read and understand that book and I said, "I don't understand this at all." I said, "I don't know why you gave it to me. I do not understand." She said, "By the end of the time, you will." And then she gave me DuBois . . . and Selye. That I understood. And she kind of worked that way with me . . . [and] I knew [she] had a personal interest in me . . . I got through my master's degree that way.

Maria described being bewildered by her inability to understand the course content and how the teacher directed her quest for insight, connecting with her by providing both encouragement—"By the end of the time, you will"— and challenge—"Read these before you come back next week." Accompanying Maria as she learned to read and under-stand difficult texts, the teacher attended to Maria's learning by being open to her questions and frustration. In other words, Maria's narrative illuminates the Concernful Practice of *Presencing: Attending and Being Open* (Diekelmann, 1995). The teacher Maria describes becomes en-gaged in Maria's struggle to learn, attending to Maria's need to "do some background work." By being open to Maria's questions, the teacher in-volved herself in Maria's struggle, involvement that Maria described as "a personal interest in me." The teacher's expertise in this practice of presencing is visible in her ability to sustain the student's interest as they work together to find texts that resonate for the student. The practice of presencing attends to learning—to letting learn (Heidegger, 1954/ 1967). If the teacher had not been skilled in this kind of practice, Maria could have become overwhelmed or discouraged or unsuccessful in the program. The teacher searches with Maria for a place of understanding from which learning can progress, and together they create a place for learning and only learning (Diekelmann, 2001) to occur.

Thus, Maria's narrative also illuminates the Concernful Practice of *Creating Places: Keeping Open a Future of Possibilities* (Diekelmann,

1995). The teacher Maria describes embraced Maria's confusion and exuded confidence that an understanding of course content could be anticipated. The teacher helped Maria recognize that confusion is not a dead end or a deficit but an experience of learning. Thus, rather than evaluating or judging Maria's knowledge as deficient, the teacher was open to Maria's struggle to learn and kept open the future of possibilities for Maria in nursing education. Similarly, Maria, rather than giving up because she had "no concept of what [the teacher] was saying," persisted and became engaged in reading, searching with the teacher for a place for understanding, keeping open the future of possibilities for the teacher. Thus, Maria's narrative illuminates how through *Creating Places: Keeping Open a Future of Possibilities* teachers and students gather to become engaged in learning.

Students interviewed in the Scandinavian study also described situations wherein they experienced the need for openness to their lifeworld. Students who enter nursing education may carry with them a natural caring attitude upon which teachers can build. Examples of basic values that are a part of students' natural caring attitude are the aim to create security, nearness, and compassion in relation to the patient. Those values are, of course, emphasized in nursing education, but the theoretical knowledge has the character of "standards," which neglects their natural caring attitude. The theoretical knowledge is taught as "lifeless" dogmas rather than experienced as encounters. Students in this study could not identify teachers' efforts to encounter them in their lifeworlds and therefore the students refused the theoretical knowledge in favor of "common sense" and the unreflective emotional capacity that rules the natural caring attitude. Students found that teachers often disseminated knowledge and theory of caring that was acontextual, too abstract, or not linked to actual practice situations. The students were then expected to apply the theoretical knowledge in practice settings. According to the students' narratives, this led to experiences of failure, insufficiency, and disappointment when they did not succeed in achieving the kind of caring practice the theory prescribed.

Similarly, in the U.S. studies, many students described experiencing learning encounters marked by the demand to apply theoretical content in practice situations. While some students were able to successfully apply caring theories in practice situations in meaningful ways, for others such encounters were "stressful" experiences. Davonte, a baccalaureate student in a senior medical-surgical course, described his experience of being assigned to a surgical intensive care unit (SICU).

I was really worried about all the equipment and all the physiology and patho [pathophysiology] I had to apply, especially when you are taught the norms but you never, never, never see the norms. That is the problem with all the stuff we are taught in class. The books and journals don't agree, and then the docs have to sort out which one they are going to pay attention to and what they want and I'm expected to know that . . . And of course my nursing [classroom] instructor wants me to put down the one right answer to every question but my clinical instructor keeps saying, "Well, it all depends." Or she tells me about times that what you thought should have happened didn't happen. It's really stressful and I feel like I am caught between these two worlds and really . . . why should we be so stressed out? If the teachers care about us why don't they work together better or try to teach us in ways that help us with things like this instead of each arguing for their own position and then we get caught in the middle. And this is supposed to be a caring profession! There have to be better ways to learn nursing than this!

Davonte's experience reveals his vulnerability and his inability to comply with the demand to apply theories he is learning in the classroom to the care he is expected to provide in the SICU. Noticeably absent in Davonte's account is the caring he provided to the assigned patients. Rather, he worries about "the equipment and all the physiology and patho" and focuses on the struggle to ascertain how to determine the "one right answer" in a context in which "it all depends." Davonte's experience challenges the underlying assumption of a direct and corresponding relationship between theory and practice that is common in nursing education. As lived, he experiences the expectation to apply theory in practice as stressful, risky, and uncaring.

Similarly, Davonte experiences his teachers as "arguing their position" rather than attending to his needs to learn nursing practice. He notices that his teachers do not care about his learning experiences despite the fact that they know he is entering a caring profession. He describes the tension this creates as being "caught between two worlds."

Reflection

Pedagogic reflection is an old idea and can be defined and interpreted in different ways (e.g., Dewey, 1933; Boud, Keogh, & Walker, 1985; Janic, 1991; Mezirow, 1991; Schön, 1995; Bengtsson, 1998). In

Lifeworld Pedagogy, reflection is understood as an act of embodied consciousness wherein one ponders not just the experience itself but also the meanings and significances of the experience and the emotions and other aspects of the lived world accompanying the experience. Reflection, therefore, always already occurs in a historical, tradition-bound, and sociocultural context and against a background of lived meaning (Gadamer, 1996). In the pedagogic situation, the matter for reflection always already includes the student, teacher, and the learning situation replete with its complexities, nuances, and lived meaning.

Because reflection involves pondering the meanings and significances of experience, it involves stepping back from the situation and considering different perspectives on it, such as what went wrong, what was confusing, and so forth. Thus, in Lifeworld Pedagogy reflection is understood against an epistemology in which reflection is inherently intentional. When we experience something it is always also experienced *as* something, that is, as something that has meaning for us. Consequently, in order to understand reflection we have to begin in the assumption that we understand the meaning of the things that we use and that we see around us as the things that belong to and signify our world (Husserl, 1936/1970). Reflection is grounded in the relationship between a person and her or his object of learning. In general, we take for granted what we see or do and we are not critical of what we perceive. In the moment of perceiving we experience the world in an all-at-once way, implicitly understanding what it means (Dahlberg & Dahlberg, 2002). In trying to understand learning, we have to begin here, in the natural attitude of perception through which we experience the world around us. No particular learning theories are required to explain this understanding. Exploring the phenomenon of learning begins with the primordial dynamic relationship between the person and the world, and what teachers do is deliberately examine that dynamic. In other words, we must avoid treating as static a process that is inherently dynamic to pursue a more complex understanding of the dynamic itself.

Reflection in a phenomenology of learning and teaching involves an awareness of the need to develop a reflective lifeworld-oriented stance through the use of narratives. Lifeworld Pedagogy melds reflection with caring-science education to enrich the experience of learning in nursing as well as learning in other healthcare practices.

This pursuit is the core of teaching. The teacher, using Lifeworld

Pedagogy and listening to a learner's narrative, seeks to grasp the learner's experience in trying to understand something, in attempting to see in a different way from before the learning experience (Marton, 1986; Marton, Watkins, & Tang, 1997). Likewise, in the context of Narrative Pedagogy, learning reveals itself as new understandings that keep open a future of new possibilities. In the use of phenomenological pedagogies, then, teaching is undergoing a transformation wherein disciplinary knowledge is intrawoven with experience. In both pedagogies described here, teaching and learning shape and are shaped by teachers and students mindfully listening to and engaging themselves in the learning encounter.

Thought of in this way, teaching is by no means anything teachers add or bring to the learning situation. Teachers enacting Narrative Pedagogy or Lifeworld Pedagogy do not practice a certain "Method" or "Technique." Rather, they enact these pedagogies by staying engaged in the learning situation through listening and attending to students. The important thing teachers do that does not belong to the natural attitude is to take a critical stance and attempt to see what is happening when the learner grapples with understanding something in a new way. While the learner may consistently be in a natural attitude, the teacher is not. On the contrary, in order to support the learner's understanding the teacher must adopt a reflective and critical stance, one that systematically analyzes the experience of the learner as well as the teacher's own experience of the situation.

However, it is not the case that the teacher enacting a phenomenological pedagogy uses "nothing." But any strategy the teacher uses in the learning encounter arises from the encounter and cannot be decided on beforehand. Instead, the teacher is present with the learner in the encounter and practices the phenomenological, epistemological principles of openness (see Dahlberg et al., 2001).

In the U.S. studies, teachers enacted Narrative Pedagogy in their classrooms as a way of gathering students to reflect on nursing practice. Tia, an experienced teacher of undergraduate students, shares how she encourages reflection in her post-clinical conferences. She gives students a short, reflective writing assignment and then asks them to read what they have written to the group. As the teacher, Tia does the assignment too. In this way, she enacts Narrative Pedagogy by guiding beginning students in how to practice reflection in the context of clinical practice.

I do post-conference after every clinical and . . . at the beginning of the semester, because I'm working with beginning students that are so excited about every new thing they do, I just let them recount their day and they say, "Oh today I . . ." And that's ok because I pull out of that, you know, like, "So what were you thinking at this point?" Or, "How did you come to that conclusion?" And that's fine but when you get to a certain point in the semester they're not as interested, you know, they've all done injections, all that stuff so that the skills that are initially REAL exciting to them aren't any more and you want to get them into thinking about different things. So I started passing this sheet around with a bunch of phrases on it. I have a student pick one and then we all take 5–10 minutes and write about it. And then . . . we all read what we have written . . . and we all chime in and talk about the experience. This last time a student picked the phrase, "Today I wondered about . . ." And so they all wrote and when they read their stuff . . . it was like, "Oh my gosh, [as a teacher] I never realized these kinds of things were going on in their [the students'] heads!" You THINK you know what they're thinking because you know where you WANT them to think but that isn't what happened. After they told me what they wondered about then it got ME to wonder how they got to thinking in that way, it was like, "WOW, how did they get here?"

At the beginning of the term, Tia gives her beginning students time to talk about the new skills they are learning and practicing in the clinical situation. Although these discussions tend to be a "recounting" of the day's activities, Tia asks the students questions like "So what were you thinking at that point?" to assist students in beginning to see complexity in their practice. When the students become experienced enough that they are no longer interested in or challenged by this approach, Tia assembles a list of open-ended phrases such as: "Today I wondered about . . . ," "Today I was worried when . . . ," and "I was surprised when . . ." to prompt them to "think about different things." In this way Tia encourages the students to reflect on their practice and compels them to think together about their practice as more than a constellation of new skills.

When Tia enacts Narrative Pedagogy by gathering students to reflect on their practice, she creates a place for both teacher and students to think about nursing practice "differently." Tia's approach is based on the mption that Narrative Pedagogy begins with teachers and students reflecting on and sharing their lived experiences and challenging the self-evident assumptions in their practice, which Tia describes as "You THINK you know what [students] are thinking because you know where you WANT them to think." Although Tia is an experienced clinical teacher, when she and her students share their experiences she is "surprised" by students' thinking and wonders "how did they get here?"

However, developing new pedagogies—substantively revising how we, as teachers, think about teaching and learning—is risky. Traditionally, concern over students' abilities to provide (nursing) care has caused many teachers to try to teach more content and skills. For instance, some teachers described either "giving up" on meeting with students following clinical experiences so that students "don't miss anything out on the [clinical] unit" or using post-clinical time to "provide more material." Using post-clinical time having students either amass more content knowledge or perform more practical skills and interventions inadvertently reproduces conventional pedagogies. In both cases the result is an additive curriculum (Diekelmann et al., 1989). The assumption that goes unchallenged is that teaching content is central to learning nursing practice because without content, students will have no foundation or basis for their thinking. In this case, thinking is considered to be the application of content or skills to a particular situation. Thinking follows learning skills and content. It is this deeply held assumption that results in an inordinate amount of emphasis being placed on learning new content and skills in both classroom and clinical courses. The additive curriculum is endemic in conventional nursing education.

The stories shared by teachers and students in these studies reflect the influence of the additive curriculum on the day-to-day lives of both students and teachers. Teachers described spending more and more time teaching content and skills and students described spending more and more time attempting to assimilate and demonstrate their mastery of new information and skills to the point where both students and teachers realized there was no time for thinking or collectively reflecting on practice.

In the Scandinavian study, students' descriptions of their learning experiences explicated how reflection has the power to fuse students' lifeworlds with caring-science knowledge. Such an understanding of reflection means a kind of coalescence of theoretical knowledge, life experience, and caring experience, similar to what Gadamer (1995) describes as a "fusion of horizons." The coalescence occurs gradually and in a symbolic way. It can be understood as the development of a personal caring-science paradigm. It is a process that requires pedagogies that allow enough silence and, most important, time for reflection—as one student said, "It takes time for the caring theory to sink into oneself." A coalescence of knowledge and experience is achieved via reflection, meaning that every caregiver is a bearer of caring-scientific knowledge, which is a vital knowledge that includes several dimensions of learning, such as language and acting. The students characterized this coalescence as "the caring theory is integrated in my being as a caregiver" or as "my caring-theoretical approach is integrated in me, I act like that every day."

Students in the master's program described this coalescence as deeply rooted and argued that it was difficult to discern the caring-theoretical structure in their approach to caring in general. The more the caring-science theory was integrated in the lifeworld of students, the more holistic the caring approach became. The fusion of life paradigm and caring-science paradigm occurred through a new form of natural attitude: "it is about this caring approach, *my* approach." Because this new form of natural attitude is based on reflective awareness, it is more solid than the "old" natural attitude, based on common sense:

As with reflection, I mean, that you never do anything automatically, but think it over . . . you never do something just as routine.

In order to develop this caring attitude the student must acquire a core of caring-science theory and experience practicing (and reflecting on practice) in a caring way. This caring attitude enables the student to relate to the individual patient's lifeworld and prevents routinized or oppressive behavior in caring contexts.

Conventional approaches inadvertently reinforce the separation or the distinction between practical and theoretical knowledge, often described as a "gap" or "breach" (Alexander, 1983; Benner, 1984; McCaugherty, 1991; Pilhammar-Andersson, 1993; Rolfe, 1996; Rooke, 1991; Sandin, 1988) between caring practice and praxis. That is, teachers base their practice of teaching on the idea that having students amass more content knowledge best prepares them to practice nursing. Simi-larly, other teachers privilege practical knowledge, adding more clinical hours to their courses. This approach is based on the assumption that ɔtudent who has performed the greatest number of skills is better prepared to practice nursing. In both these cases the nature of relationship between practical and theoretical knowledge is left unconsidered. That is, these approaches privilege either practical knowledge (more practice time) or theoretical knowledge (more content).

What is missing is what Heidegger refers to as the between or the space that gathers, in this case, the theoretical and the practical. The task for thinking, Heidegger contends, is not to attend to one over the other, nor to both together, but to the between, the thinking that is simultaneously both and neither theoretical nor practical. Following this path to thinking requires the recognition that the between is not the space which joins the practical and the theoretical. Rather, Heidegger (1927/1962) describes the between as that which reaches beyond and back behind our categorization of thinking. The task for thinking, then, is to ponder not the different kinds of knowledge but how practical and theoretical knowledge belong together. So the question becomes, how do teachers teach thinking in the between?

To teach the between requires that simple causal models of thinking, which Hillocks (1999) refers to as "if-then" models, be overcome. If-then models are evident in the assumption that *if* students are provided with "enough material" *then* they will be able to apply that knowledge in providing care to patients. This if-then model of teaching is deeply embedded in conventional approaches to, for example, nursing education. It is frequently assumed that beginning students require such models to safely enter healthcare (or, caring) practice. We are not arguing that teachers should never teach content, or never have students complete case studies or spend additional time in a clinical setting. We are too experienced in nursing education to succumb to such a shortsighted and simplistic solution. Rather, what we have learned from research in nursing education is that teachers around the world are creating new pedagogies and substantively new ways to do things differently by giving up on the idea that we can keep doing "what we currently do" if we just do it better. Sometimes these changes are small but end up having a profound impact on teaching and learning.

Phenomenological pedagogies mark a shift away from the conventional if-then assumptions in teaching students to provide care that prespecifies and anticipates what the learning and thinking will be in practice situations. Even in approaches such as the one the Scandinavian study presented here documents, where caring-science substance is central to nursing education, we want to emphasize that significant learning arises out of lived situations when teachers are open to the students' lifeworlds and reflect on the meanings and significances of their learning encounters.

The Learning Communion and Community Practices

In our analysis of Narrative Pedagogy and Lifeworld Pedagogy we found a common emphasis on the learning communion that occurs between and among students and teachers or the community practices of learning. In phenomenological pedagogies the learning encounter is marked by efforts to overcome teacher-centeredness by creating new partnerships between and among students and teachers.

In Lifeworld Pedagogy, these new partnerships revolve around the personal (not private) relationship between a teacher and a student. The term *learning communion* refers to this relationship, which is constituted by nearness, openness, and sensitivity to the other. In Narrative Pedagogy, new partnerships are community experiences in which teachers and students gather to collectively seek new understandings in the context of nursing education and practice. The term *community practices* reflects the commitment to privilege neither the individual teacher or student nor the group, but to create learning environments that are inclusive and collective. Thus, in Narrative Pedagogy, caring is a community practice that students and teachers co-create in their learning encounters. Thus, *engendering community*, or the reciprocity of caring between and among students and teachers, is central in the enacting of Narrative Pedagogy.

In the context of phenomenological pedagogies, the teacher accompanies students in learning, providing opportunities for them to extend, enhance, and critique their understandings of caring, rather than being the arbiter of course discussions. This does not mean that the teacher provides the students with no guidance, support, or direction. On the contrary, it means that the teacher is working with students to help them safely enter practice, posing questions of how, what, and why for the students' reflection.

The Scandinavian research shows how students experience a caring, learning communion (that allows a reflective approach in relation to the phenomenon of caring). The students are also supported by the teacher in their struggles to balance "nearness" and "distance" in relation to patients' suffering and well-being. This study demonstrates how important learning communion is in relation to caring situations, particularly those that demand the "courage to come close." Learning communion is strengthened by the fact that the teacher is a "genuine carrier of caring culture." One graduate student in the Scandinavian study expressed it thus:

The best teacher is the excellent nurse who has an integrated caring approach, she lives the caring science. Students should meet that kind of person very early in the nursing education.

Another graduate student in the Scandinavian project talked about the need for teachers to practice openness and uniqueness:

You need to use concepts that the student understands and that she can relate to her own experiences and world. Because you must call for their own subjective experiences . . . , otherwise it does not work. You cannot teach about examples of experiences that the student does not have.

A didactic challenge for teachers is to interact with students within the learning encounter in ways that support and enhance student learning. Different approaches make abstract theoretical substance vital— for example, the use of narratives, paintings, or drama exercises. In a recent supervision project (Lepp et al., 2001) it was found that role-playing had a vivifying effect on the understanding of theoretical structures. Teaching approaches that encourage thinking, feeling, and acting help students experience caring knowledge in a creative way, with all their senses. Furthermore, individual encounters in small groups allow for the creation of individually adapted didactics and a learning relationship that is characterized by nearness, openness, and sensitivity. The Scandinavian research concludes that in large groups neither students nor teachers experience good didactic relationships. Thus, large groups may prevent rather than promote learning.

Students who experience caring science as vital trust the knowledge they acquire and may, as a consequence, develop a sense of security in the learning situation. In addition, the teacher's attitude of openness toward the student's lifeworld, in combination with a solid and sound caring-science background, becomes an ideal for the student, who likewise wants to enable such vivid encounters with patients. Lifeworld Pedagogy, with its open and reflective approach to caring science in nursing education, optimizes the possibility of the student nurse to develop an open and reflective approach to patients and colleagues.

The student is dependent on the teacher's awareness of the pedagogical influence and meaning of the lifeworld perspective. Teachers must be mindful, however, of students becoming too dependent on them. The students are vulnerable in this respect, especially since they know that soon they will be on their own and encounter a complex caring reality. As one student stated:

you need to stay on and think, what actually is there, you need to be flexible and able to think in different ways . . . and also need to have a chance to practice how it is to take responsibility and act in an independent way.

The students know that after the education they have to begin "in the caring reality." They cannot begin in an ideal situation that does not exist.

In the U.S. studies, teachers enacted Narrative Pedagogy in their classrooms as a way of gathering students together to think about nursing practice. Tia, whose experience enacting Narrative Pedagogy in the post-clinical conference was recounted above, describes how she challenges students to think about their practice differently and to collectively make sense of their knowledge and experiences in clinical situations.

As each student reads, something magical happens. Like the other day, one student started with, "Today I wondered when I was going to get to sit down" . . . Another student wondered about a lab test for her patient . . . [because she] couldn't figure out what it was for . . . One student wondered when her client would really go home because he was being told he was going to a nursing home to extend his recovery time . . . and she thought we were lying to him. She thought that was just a way nurses were getting him out of the hospital and that he was really going there to die. So that led to a discussion for all of us . . . about the healthcare system because she was really distrusting the whole system . . . and I was really happy that she was able to say that and . . . to have us talk about it . . . And we just got into this big discussion about healthcare and how it's changed and I've never had that with beginning students . . . Another student shared that she wondered when she would get through a day and not forget anything. And it was like, "Oh my gosh, that's what I'm wondering too!" What I've noticed is at this point in the semester they're forgetting the things we did the very first week, like charting I&Os [intake and output]. And I had always interpreted that as, "You guys are getting sloppy, what's the matter with you?" And as she read her reflections I heard her tell how I had pointed out to her, "You forgot to chart your 2:00 I&O" and she hadn't forgotten to chart it in her mind, because that day she had hung a piggy back and a new IV bag and this was her very first time to do that and record it on the I&O sheet. She remembered that she had to do it instead of ME reminding her and so for her it was a glorious day—she had picked up something new and remembered what she had to do. But in my mind she had forgotten a basic thing. But when I heard her read it was like, "Wait a minute Tia, you're being too hard on these students. They're working so hard to add new things on that they focus on what's new and forget the old. It's not that they're lazy, it's that they are working so hard to do it right and to remember it all without me reminding them." And it just made me think differently about this pattern and I've seen this pattern every semester. I've always thought they were getting lazy [at the end of the semester]!

Tia provides these beginning students with time to practice thinking as a community experience. This challenges the conventional approach whereby a student's thinking is a personal and private experience that the teacher evaluates. Here, when both teacher and students describe their experience, they illuminate how they are making sense of or interpreting their experiences, since even the details that are included in writing involve an interpretation of that experience. By exploring with students how clinical situations are interpreted, teachers show how theoretical thinking and practical thinking become seamlessly intrawoven. For instance, when a student wonders, "are we are telling patients the truth?" she challenges a taken-for-granted practice in nursing by providing an alternative interpretation of a clinical experience and by creating a place for the community to think together about their practice.

Tia describes exploring how students interpret their experiences as "magical." When Tia states, "I've never had that with beginning students," she speaks to a common assumption of conventional approaches to education—that information is best processed by starting with the simple and moving to the complex. Tia relates how a beginning student challenges the veracity of the healthcare system and raises concern about decisions that appear to be based on economic considerations rather than on the patient's need for care even before the student is presented with such topics in a course typically taught at the senior level. This beginning student's insight and concern propelled the discussion beyond content about the healthcare system, reimbursement, and patient outcomes and reflects a situated, embodied interpretation of current practice.

Notice that Tia's story does not provide the answer to the question of veracity in this situation. Rather, the emphasis is on the teacher and students learning to interpret situations by writing, reading, and discussing their thinking. Tia's enactment of Narrative Pedagogy encourages her students to think about how clinical situations are interpreted or understood. Tia teaches the students to interpret situations as she explores with them their shared experiences of clinical practice. For example, when Tia hears students' thinking from the "inside-out" she finds that how she has been interpreting their "outside-in" comportment is not right. As a teacher, she learns, "It's not that they're lazy, it's that they're working so hard."

Tia's narrative, which shows how she provides time during post-clinical conferences to assist students in learning how to interpret by engaging in writing, illuminates the Concernful Practice of *Preserving: Reading, Writing, Thinking, and Dialogue*. The writing, in this case, is not a mere recording of experiences. Rather, to complete the selected phrase students must reflect on and interpret their experiences. Thinking of it in this way, writing is an interpretive practice of thinking:

I have them write because it really makes them think, and it really makes ME think because you don't know what you are going to get and [as a teacher] you need time to reflect on your day and you get this phrase and it makes you think about what WAS I thinking about today, what DID worry me today because . . . it's at the end of the day and you're just thinking "WHEW, I got through another day!" And I know the students are thinking the same thing. But when they write then you can really see everybody's really working at . . . thinking about their day . . . Writing seems to help them organize and express their thoughts and it insures that, as a group, we give time to and respect each other's thinking rather than all of our experiences being shaped by what the first person says . . . Writing it helps them get their head into reflecting on their day—to relive their day and give voice to the thoughts going around in their heads. It's a simple thing, really. I give 5–10 minutes at the beginning of post clinical to write and then we all read our reflections to each other and the dialogue that follows is just unbelievable! And I'm always amazed at the things that are going on in their heads that I NEVER realized they were thinking about.

By building time into post-clinical conferences for reflective writing and reading, Tia encourages students to think and engenders a community in which to practice thinking. Thinking in nursing practice is both an individual and a community practice (Benner et al., 1996), and Tia's approach provokes students to think in ways that parallel what it will be like for them when they enter practice:

Like, when the student said she wondered when she would get to sit down. I don't think a student would have said that to a teacher, but when you're in the moment, then they share how they experienced their clinical time. So when the student said, I wonder when I would get to sit down, several other students jumped in and shared what a hard day it was, and how many days in clinical they don't get to sit down, and how hard it is to never get that down time. So she got supported from her colleagues in a different way than had she not shared it with us.

Conventional approaches often privilege writing that demonstrates the correct matching of patient problems with interventions or the correct application of theoretical knowledge to a practical problem. Tia enacts Narrative Pedagogy by asking students to write as a means of encouraging thinking, which may be both, or neither, practical or theoretical. Also embedded in Tia's description is the seamlessness of reading, writing, thinking, and dialogue as practices that co-occur in learning situations. For instance, students "organize and express their thoughts" in writing but "give voice" to their thoughts by reading their reflections aloud to the group. That is, as students' thoughts are committed to paper, thinking becomes visible, and reading aloud draws the group into a dialogue that articulates, revises, and challenges their understanding of nursing practice. In this way, Tia demonstrates that preserving the belongingness among reading, writing, thinking, and dialogue is vital to learning nursing practice in this beginning clinical course.

Toward a Science of Education for Health Professions

The phenomenological pedagogies presented here grew out of nursing research for nursing education and, as such, contribute to and extend the science of nursing education. Enacting these pedagogies enables students and teachers to develop new insights into the substance of nursing knowledge (emphasizing caring science) in relation to the patient for whom care is provided. The new understandings and insights gleaned from enacting these pedagogies also enhance the substance of nursing or caring-science knowledge. Nursing and other caring epistemologies are augmented by teachers' openness to the students' lifeworld, by the analysis of caring (nursing) narratives in pedagogical situations, and by the new understandings that are created between and among teachers and students in the context of praxis. Thus, discovering new understandings of practice can be theory generating (Benner et al., 1996).

To enact a phenomenological pedagogy is to insure that teachers don't become the center and measure of all learning. Such an approach, which includes encouraging the students involved in learning to make use of narratives, also prevents nursing education or other health profession education from being reduced to skills, strategies, or "mere utility." Enacting a phenomenological pedagogy shifts the focus from teaching to learning and is student-oriented rather than teacher-oriented.

Lifeworld Pedagogy contributes to the general understanding of a phenomenological pedagogy with its emphasis on the idea of going "back to the things themselves." In this case, the "things themselves" are the learners, their lifeworld, their narratives, and their approach to learning, teaching, and schooling, which shapes and informs the pedagogy. This phenomenology of learning is not a new technique; it is not a new set of technologies or strategies. Instead it is "a rediscovery of what already is and as such it is simple, familiar, and at hand" (Diekelmann & Diekelmann, 2000, p. 230). One could say that enacting a phenomenological pedagogy is to go on living and experiencing as we do everyday, but in a slower, more systematic, more methodical, and more reflective way. Teachers using this approach, however, need to be more open and sensitive to the phenomena (the students and the learning encounter) and their way of presenting themselves than is necessary in "the natural attitude" in which we commonly live our lives as teachers.

Lifeworld encounters and the understanding of narratives within the context of caring-science education are shaped by the caring-science substance; that is, caring science "perspectivizes" the understanding of learning and teaching. The pedagogy of caring science is to be understood as the art of learning and teaching within the framework of caring science, which means that caring-science pedagogy is based on the same ontological foundation as the rest of caring science. The pedagogy of caring science is a subdiscipline of caring science, and is thus contextually dependant on the caring-science perspective. Central assumptions of caring science, such as an explicit attention to the patient's perspective, with an emphasis on her or his suffering and wellness, are consequently reflected in the encounter between learners and teachers (Eriksson, 1987, 1993) and in subsequent encounters in which nurses participate in, and come to know and understand, the patient's lifeworld (her or his experiences and narratives of health, illness, suffering, wellness, and care). Further, such a pedagogy also affects the substance of caring science in that the caring science will change and grow as a result of the narratives and the dynamics in general within the lifeworld approach.

To summarize, then, a central concern of the Lifeworld Pedagogy is attending to the lifeworld of the learners; beginning with the lived experience and the notion of reflection, the natural attitude is enriched and perspectivized by caring science, which supports students' growth in a personal as well as a professional sense.

Narrative Pedagogy contributes to the general understanding of phenomenological pedagogies in being a way of thinking and a community practice that gathers phenomenological, critical, and feminist pedagogies along with postmodern discourses to create new possibilities for schooling, learning, and teaching. The shared experiences of students, teachers, and clinicians are described as *The Concernful Practices of Schooling, Learning, and Teaching*. These practices also provide a new language for contemporary health professions education. Teachers, students, and clinicians cannot escape or overcome the metaphysical claims of language, but they can seek new understandings that may illuminate neoteric possibilities for health professions education. Narrative Pedagogy encourages teachers and students to pause, to ponder, to hold open and problematic the commitments the language of schooling, learning, and teaching make in our scientific epoch (modern epoch). The Concernful Practices provide a common, nontechnical and nonscientific description of schooling, learning, and teaching that arises from within the community but that is simultaneously a part of the scientific and technical community.

Attending to history is a central concern of Narrative Pedagogy. Students, teachers, and clinicians commonly tell of old traditions and practices they found meaningful and helpful that are now lost, forgotten, or overlooked. Yet the recuperation of these traditions does not represent a romantic return to a previous kind of schooling; rather this recuperation demonstrates the ongoing process of preserving and extending the shared practices of human comportment in the context of schooling, learning, and teaching.

Narrative Pedagogy is committed to a discourse that describes the wisdom and practical knowledge gained through experience in schooling, learning, and teaching (Benner et al., 1996). In explicating narratives, teachers and students embrace the insights of science and a rational approach to understanding schooling, learning, and teaching while also critiquing their objectification of schooling, learning, and teaching and use of a will-to-will (Heidegger 1927/1962) or power. For instance, in the context of health professions education, is the only kind of learning that is valued that which relates directly to interventions (the goal of practice being to intervene in patient situations) or is interpretive inquiry valued and encouraged as well? What does our language and practice assume (or overlook) about how students, teachers, or clinicians understand (or don't understand) a patient's situation or experience (Ironside et al., in press)?

Similarly, teachers and students are able to glean insights from shared experiences that reveal the practical wisdom and knowledge of schooling, learning, and teaching. These shared practices are also critiqued for privileging language and experience and for using and abusing language as power.

Teachers and students also explore the background practices that are revealed through their descriptions of schooling, learning, and teaching experiences. In producing interpretations and explications of these shared experiences (The Concernful Practices of Schooling, Learning, and Teaching), teachers and students move toward embracing an interpretive scholarship that reveals the constitutive nature of schooling, learning, and teaching. This pedagogical approach encourages teachers and students to explore their common experiences and their shared meanings in the context of schooling, learning, and teaching.

This elucidation of a phenomenological pedagogy, including commonalities of and differences between the Lifeworld Pedagogy and the Narrative Pedagogy, is a first step toward a science of education for health professions. The science of education in the health professions is enriched and extended when teachers and students reflect on the commitments and assumptions embedded in discipline-specific neoteric approaches to education (Ironside, 2001). As new pedagogies are developed from health professions research for health professions education, continuing research is needed to ascertain the meaningfulness of these approaches in various disciplinary contexts and to explore the promise that is embedded in each approach for meeting the contemporary challenges of practice education. Discipline-specific pedagogies take advantage of and also extend pedagogical approaches that have been developed in other disciplines. In other words, merely importing educational theories that are frequently more academic than practical (Ironside, 2001) into health professions education overlooks the contingencies of practice and the contemporary context of healthcare that influence the health science disciplines. Without creating, implementing, and evaluating new pedagogies in specific disciplinary contexts the practice of teaching the health professions will be based on anecdotal evidence (or trial and error) rather than on evidence produced by rigorous research (Ironside, 2002).

Furthermore, creating discipline-specific pedagogies contributes to a science of health professions education. Without a cadre of researchers systematically studying discipline-specific pedagogies, all research related to how the health science professions are taught and learned will be carried out in schools of education or will be done by healthcare providers using theories from disciplines committed to studying teaching and learning. The danger in this strategy (other than the obvious one that it will fail to account for the contingencies of contemporary practice) is that the pedagogical approach used in schools of nursing, for instance, in essence shapes or structures the discipline. New nurses (or other health professionals) learn what matters in the discipline by how they experience their educational preparation. The students in both the U.S. and Scandinavian studies experienced the dissonance of attempting to learn caring practice in an uncaring environment. Developing discipline-specific pedagogies insures we are "walking the talk" of educational reform.

Enacting a phenomenological pedagogy calls on students and teachers to persistently consider what is meaningful in the experience of education that should be preserved and extended, as well as what is not meaningful or what is oppressive and should be overcome or abolished. In this way health professions education can remain responsive to the changing milieu of healthcare, and to the evolving knowledge (and ways of knowing) and experience of community members.

Faced with rapidly changing and economically stressed international healthcare systems, the growing diversity among teachers and students (as well as among recipients of care), the teacher shortage, and the increasing demand for, and the mounting demands placed on, new health professionals, the need to develop research-based approaches to health professions education has never been greater. In such chaotic times, teachers and students might be tempted to either hold on tight to conventional and familiar approaches because they provide a sense of security or to discard any approach that is not considered novel or unique because it appears to offer no promise. Similarly, it is easy to trivialize any substantive alternative as "lowering the standards" of an idealized notion of education in the absence of systematic evaluative data on which to base such claims. Perhaps the challenge for teachers and students is to persistently seek to understand which practices to hold on tight to and which to discard as they extend conventional pedagogical practices through creating new research-based, discipline-specific pedagogies. That is, perhaps it is by teachers and students continually and tenaciously questioning and exploring the practices of schooling, learning, and teaching that new possibilities for health professions education will emerge.

Presented in part to the National League for Nursing Convention, Miami, FL.

References

Alexander, M. F. (1983). *Learning to nurse: Integrating theory and practice*. Edinburgh: Churchill Livingstone.

Andrews, C. A., Ironside, P. M., Nosek, C., Sims, S. L., Swenson, M. M., Yeomans, C., Young, P. K., & Diekelmann, N. L. (2001). Enacting narrative pedagogy: The lived experiences of students and teachers. *Nursing and Health Care Perspectives, 22*(5), 252–259.

Bengtsson, J. (1998). *Fenomenologiska utflykter* (Phenomenological excursions). Göteborg: Daidalos.

Benner, P. (1984). *From novice to expert. Excellence and power in clinical nursing practice*. Menlo Park, CA: Addison-Wesley.

Benner, P., Tanner, C., & Chesla, C. A. (1996). *Expertise in nursing practice: Caring, clinical judgment, and ethics*. New York: Springer.

Boud, D., Keogh, R., & Walker, D. (Eds.). (1985). *Reflection: Turning experience into learning*. London: Kogan Page Ltd.

Dahlberg, H., & Dahlberg, K. (2002). *To not make definite what is indefinite: A phenomenological analysis of perception and its epistemological consequences in human science research*. Paper presented at the 21st International Human Science Research Conference, Victoria, Canada.

Dahlberg, K., Drew, N., & Nyström, M. (2001). *Reflective lifeworld research*. Lund: Studentlitteratur.

Dewey, J. (1933). *How we think. A restatement of the relation of reflective thinking to the educative process*. Boston: D. C. Heath.

Diekelmann, N. (1995). Reawakening thinking: Is traditional pedagogy nearing completion? *Journal of Nursing Education, 34*(5), 195–196.

Diekelmann, N. (2001). Narrative pedagogy: Heideggerian hermeneutical analyses of lived experiences of students, teachers, and clinicians. *Advances in Nursing Science, 23*(3), 53–71.

Diekelmann, N., Allen, D., & Tanner, C. (1989). *The National League for Nursing criteria for appraisal of baccalaureate programs: A critical hermeneutic analysis*. New York: National League for Nursing Press.

Diekelmann, N., & Diekelmann, J. (2000). Learning ethics in nursing and genetics: Narrative Pedagogy and the grounding of values. *Journal of Pediatric Nursing, 15*(4), 226–231.

Diekelmann, N., & Diekelmann, J. (forthcoming). *Schooling learning teaching: Toward a Narrative Pedagogy*. Madison: University of Wisconsin Press.

Diekelmann, N., & Ironside, P. (1998a). Hermeneutics. In J. Fitzpatrick (Ed.), *Encyclopedia of Nursing Research*. New York: Springer.

Diekelmann, N., & Ironside, P. (1998b). Preserving writing in doctoral education: Exploring the concernful practices of schooling learning teaching. *Journal of Advanced Nursing, 28*(6), 1347–1355.

Ekebergh, M. (2001). *Tillägnandet av vårdvetenskaplig kunskap—reflexionens betydelse för lärandet* (Acquiring caring science knowledge, the importance of reflection for caring). Unpublished doctoral dissertation, Åbo: Åbo Akademi.

Eriksson, K. (1987). *Vårdandets idé* (The idea of caring). Stockholm: Almqvist & Wiksell.

Eriksson, K. (1990/1984). *Hälsans idé* (The idea of health). Stockholm: Almqvist & Wiksell.

Eriksson, K. (1993). *Möten med lidande* (Encountering suffering). Rapport nr. 4, Institutionen för vårdvetenskap, Åbo Akademi: Åbo Akademis tryckeri.

Eriksson, K., & Lindström, U., (Red.). (2000). *Gryning. En vårdvetenskaplig antologi* (Dawn. A caring science anthology). Vasa: Institutionen för vårdvetenskap, Åbo Akademi.

Gadamer, H. G. (1995). *Truth and method*. (2nd rev. ed). (J. Weinsheimer & D. Marshall, Rev. Trans.). New York: Continuum. (Original German work published in 1960.)

Gadamer, H. G. (1996). *The enigma of health*. (J. Geiger and N. Walker, Trans.) Stanford, CA: Stanford University Press.

Giorgi, A. (1997). The theory, practice, and evaluation of the phenomenological method as a quality research procedure. *Journal of Phenomenological Psychology, 28*, 235–260.

Grondin, J. (1990). Hermeneutics and relativism. In K. Wright (Ed.), *Festivals of interpretation: Essays on Hans-Georg Gadamer's work*. Albany: State University of New York Press.

Heidegger, M. (1962). *Being and time*. (J. Macquarrie & E. Robinson, Trans.). New York: Harper. (Original German work published 1927.)

Heidegger, M. (1967). *What is a thing?* (W. B. Barton & V. Deutsch, Trans.). Chicago: Henry Regnery. (Original German work published 1954.)

Hillocks, G. Jr. (1999). *Ways of thinking, ways of teaching*. New York: Teachers College Press.

Husserl, E. (1970). *The crisis of European sciences and transcendental phenomenology: An introduction to phenomenological philosophy* (D. Carr, Trans.). Evanston, IL: Northwestern University Press. (Original German work published 1936.)

Ironside, P. M. (1997). *Preserving reading, writing, thinking, and dialogue: Rethinking doctoral education in nursing*. Unpublished doctoral dissertation, University of Wisconsin–Madison.

Ironside, P. M. (1999). Thinking in nursing education—Part II: A teacher's perspective. *Nursing and Health Care Perspectives, 20*(5), 243–247.

Ironside, P. M. (2001). Creating a research base for nursing education: An interpretive review of conventional, critical, feminist, postmodern, and phenomenologic pedagogies. *Advances in Nursing Science, 23*(3), 72–87.

Ironside, P. M. (2002). *Trying something new: Implementing and evaluating Narrative Pedagogy using a multi-method approach*. Manuscript submitted for publication.

Ironside, P. M., Scheckel, M., Wessels, C., Bailey, M., Powers, S., & Seeley, D. (in press). Experiencing chronic illness: Co-creating new understandings. *Journal of Qualitative Health Research*.

Janic, A. (1991). *Cordelias tysnad. Om reflexionens kunskapsteori* (The silence of Cordelia. An epistemology of relection). Stockholm: Carlssons.

Kavanagh, K. (1998). Summers of no return: Transforming care through a nursing field school. *Journal of Nursing Education, 37*(2), 71–79.

Lepp, M., Ekebergh, M., & Dahlberg, K. (2001). *The lifeworld in focus in nursing education supervision*. Paper presented at the Chicago Institute in Nursing Education Diversity in Nursing Education: Web of Challenges—Wealth of Opportunities Chicago.

MacLeod, M. L. (1996). *Practicing nursing: Becoming experienced*. Edinburgh: Churchill Livingstone.

Marton, F. (1986). Phenomenography—a research approach to investigating different understandings of reality. *Journal of Thought, 21*(3), 28–49.

Marton, F., Watkins, D., & Tang, C. (1997). Discontinuities and continuities in the experience of learning: An interview study of high-school students in Hong Kong. *Learning and Instruction, 7*(1), 21–48.

McCaugherty, D. (1991). The theory-practice gap in nursing education: Its causes and possible solutions. Findings from an action research study. *Journal of Advanced Nursing, 16*, 1055–1061.

Merleau-Ponty, M. (1995). *Phenomenology of perception*. (C. Smith, Trans.). London: Routledge. (Original French work published in 1945.)

Mezirow, J. (1991). *Transformative dimensions of adult learning*. San Francisco: Jossey-Bass.

Palmer, R. E. (1969). *Hermeneutics: Interpretation theory in Schleiermacher, Dilthey, Heidegger, and Gadamer*. Evanston, IL: Northwestern University Press.

Pilhammar Andersson, E. (1991). *Det är vi som är dom. Sjuksköterskestuderandes föreställningar och perspektiv under utbildningstiden* (Dissertation about nursing students' ideas of their education). Göteborg studies in educational sciences, nr. 83. Göteborg: Acta Universitatis Gothoburgensis.

Rolfe, G. (1996). *Closing the theory-practice gap. A new paradigm for nursing.* Oxford: Butterworth-Heinemann.

Rooke, L. (1991). *Omvårdnad–teoretiska ansatser i praktisk verksamhet* (Nursing—theoretical approaches in practice). Stockholm: Almqvist & Wiksell.

Sandin, I. (1988). *Att forskningsanknyta vårdproblem. Om mötet mellan kunskapstraditioner* (About the meeting of different traditions of knowledge in caring). Forskningsgruppen för kunskapsutveckling och pedagogik. (Rapport nr. 6). Stockholm: Stockholms universitet, pedagogiska institutionen.

Schön, D. (1995). *The reflective practitioner: How professionals think in action.* Aldershot, Hants, U. K.: Arena. (Original work published in 1983)

Swenson, M. M., & Sims, S. L. (2000). Toward a narrative-centered curriculum for family nurse practitioners. *Journal of Nursing Education, 39*(3), 109–115.

Young, P. K. (1998). *Joining the academic community: The lived experiences of new teachers in nursing education.* Unpublished doctoral dissertation, University of Wisconsin–Madison.

2

Mirrors

A Cultural and Historical Interpretation of Nursing's Pedagogies

Kathryn Hopkins Kavanagh

What we do about history matters.
Lerner, 1997, p. 204

The histories of nursing and nursing pedagogies—including the art, craft, work, and acts (Carlson & Apple, 1998), and the thinking about and comportment associated with teaching (Ironside, 2000)—mirror the social and cultural ethos of varied times and circumstances. Perhaps more than any other occupation, nursing has been shaped by social conceptions of women and their place in society. Yet it would be inadequate to examine nursing pedagogies from only that perspective because nursing's story is really many stories, reflecting as it does a confluence of the legacies of women (since caring for the sick and nursing are traditionally women's work) with those of education, science, medicine, hospitals, labor, industry, professionalism, ideological change, social process, and public imaging. Despite multiple and rapid transitions in each of those areas, one persistent, pervasive, and consequential theme emerges: nursing's self-deception regarding issues of class and gender (David, 2000). But the story of nursing is not a simple story of oppression or juxtaposed vulnerability and privilege. Part of nursing's story is that nurses are better at taking care of others than they are at advocating on behalf of themselves and their discipline.

59

The texts of any story include what is not said as well as what is (Hall, 1999). Ignoring differences between men's and women's histories distorts reality (Lerner, 1997) and, historically, not only has women's history been missing, but until recently its invisibility has seldom been challenged by historians (Schmidt & Schmidt, 1976). The fact that nurses' history, heretofore repressed as a part of women's history, is so faintly visible may say more about historians' priorities than about nurses (Hogeland, 1973; Sandercock, 1998; Symonds, 1991). But it also says that nurses have, in large part, accepted the quiet marginalization of their discipline, which, being neither seen nor heard, has had no real place of its own. Education has played a powerful role in nursing's peripheralization in society and in health care (Hall, 1999). While interest in women's schooling has been heightened by women's movements and feminist ideologies, sexism remains as nursing's most pervasive problem (Cleland, 1971; David, 2000; Spicker & Gadow, 1980). Women's history has traditionally been considered "not intellectually interesting" (Carroll, 1976, p. x). With "male" activities considered the norm (Lerner, 1997), labor historians find machinists and steelworkers more appealing than nurses (Melosh, 1982), while medical historians typically represent nurses as mere adjuncts to physicians. Nursing, arising in large part from what physicians did not want to do, has been represented as a vague negative of medicine (David, 2000) rather than as a significant enterprise in its own right.

Nursing's history confounds issues around representation. To write history as if women were less than or more than full persons amounts to not taking females seriously (Hogeland, 1973). Yet representing nurses as women with a history that stands complete and accurate but outside simple conformity to patriarchal expectations poses a heavy task. The challenge is made greater by nursing's ingenuous willingness to preserve its marginal status and to perpetuate its relative oppression. Preunderstandings of reality involve tradition embedded in language, but in nursing, the language of history often fails to connect the past with the present. My own experiences—an undergraduate semester of chronology alleged to be nursing history, graduate educations in nursing and in medical anthropology, and a dozen years of teaching in schools of nursing—provided few conceptual links between American nursing and American culture and society, either past or present, let alone as a whole. Despite efforts to make nursing's history relevant to its pedagogies and curricula (e.g., Keeling & Ramos, 1995), I more often saw the past denigrated as obsolete than respected. Nonetheless, today, after years of reliance on nurses untrained in historical methods recording histories shaped by their own experiences and interests, nursing finally has its own historians and historiography. However, it now faces the challenge of creating a viable future for itself. Only occasionally, within rare gatherings of scholars, have I heard the question: "How is it we have come to be the way we are?"[1] In response to that query, this chapter provides a cultural interpretation of the history of nursing pedagogies and the origins and nature of its constituent ideologies.

Mirrors of History

> To those in power, history has always mattered.
> Lerner, 1997, p. 202

Beyond its role as a mirror that reflects some version of what is going on in the broader social context, there has been little to draw attention to nursing. It is a relatively new field. Less than a century and a half ago in the United States, nursing either occurred within the home as a seemingly natural phenomenon that was part of women's work or it was limited to the ministrations of whatever poor unfortunates could be prevailed upon to tend to the ill in public institutions. The work of nursing was subject to neither inspection nor discipline, despite risks posed by and to persons regularly engaged in it (Kalisch & Kalisch, 1995). Although caring for the sick is a practice as old as humanity, it is no accident that nursing as it is known today has such a short history. The histories of the pedagogies and practices of nursing were woven from disparate threads of the broader culture—culture in terms of lived meanings that are not fixed but continuously contested because of social or political differences (Kleinman, 1995)—and society.

The meaningful world is a partially integrated set of social and symbolic forms that are fluid and ambiguous. Over time these generally appear as coherent and consensual. History involves attending to some pattern of dialectical, bipolar social equilibrium, but being cultural, always contains contestable images and actions. The scholar's task of unmasking the real is complicated by history's embodiment in both the material and the symbolic (Comaroff & Comaroff, 1992). The challenge becomes one of contextualizing the known fragments of human worlds and representing them without compromising their interactive situatedness or undermining their uniqueness. History is made in the interaction of realities that coexist in time and space. As Heidegger and Merleau-Ponty suggested, understanding history requires recognizing the ontological complicity between the agent and the social world. When one examines the underpinnings of social interests such as nursing's pedagogies, it is the dialectics embedded in the *making* of collective worlds that must be considered (Comaroff & Comaroff, 1992. Anthropology's ethnographic elucidation of sociocultural tensions (to reveal their historical contingencies and cultural configurations) facilitates the creation of humanistic accounts of the past that make explicit the dialectics that foster understanding. At one level, the relationships between fragments of knowing pose an interpretive challenge to critical reflection. At another, the use of historical imagination in critical history yields essential oppositional viewpoints. With reflexive contextualization, time is historicized in lieu of being merely chronologized. Although neither historian nor ethnographer can make the reader a native of another time and place, either can interpret meaningfully.

Too little attention has been paid to unintended consequences in nursing's history, to the hegemonic aspects of the culture that shaped that history, and to the ways in which both history and culture shape nursing today. Part of this neglect results from the dialectic between liberal discourse (unpacking hegemony) and the notion of civic community as the coherent identity of a group. But nursing's history also involves the exploitation, marginalization, and powerlessness associated with oppression (Peters, 1996). Nursing has both resisted and accepted the politics that have shaped its existence. For all of its ability to deal with the everyday exigencies of birthing, living, and dying, nursing often uses rose-colored lenses when it looks in the mirror. Resistance is minute, unnoticed (typically even by nurses), irresolute, and soon conceded. Most nurses accept this limited prospect as part of their role even when it means betraying themselves by going along with the masses (David, 2000). Nonviolent resistance can be easily overlooked even when it is strong (Lerner, 1997; Sandercock, 1998), but nurses have never truly organized to maximize their collective strength. Why are fewer strong students enrolling in nursing programs today? Perhaps it is simply a sign of unwillingness to put up with the traditional oppressions.

The confluence of ethnographic thinking and historical imagination is especially useful in challenging the categories used to characterize subordinate groups (Denzin, 1997). Historians are no more reliable than ethnographers when either's scholarship encounters only fragments of a cultural field. The silences and spaces that hint at "'hidden histories' situated in wider worlds of power and meaning" (Comaroff & Comaroff, 1992, p. 17) can be examined only when meaningful interconnections of events and ideas are restored. Correcting existing misrepresentations is an essential task of representation. History is written in multidimensional experiential layers. Telling the stories of nursing's pedagogies by recounting their interrelatedness risks redundancy, as the knots are tied in many places and the mirrors reflect in all directions. Such narratives reject strict chronology, since parts of stories are told as they become relevant, while other parts may show up as parts of other stories. The goal of interpretive inquiry is useful new understandings of some collective social phenomenon. It takes a keenly critical perspective and sound analyses to ensure that scholars living in worlds different from those they study do not take undue liberties.

Occupational and academic disciplines often fail to recognize their own assumptions about specific historical contexts (Nicholson, 1990). Committed to the unexamined primacy of the individual (Kleinman, 1995), Western intellectual tradition has tended to be both gender blind and gender biased (Benhabib & Cornell, 1987). Most history has been written in terms of reigns and revolutions in which women took relatively minor, if any, part. The notion of women as naturally "there" but marginal to the mainstream of "real" history suggests that they merit notice only when they intrude upon human drama in unnatural ways (Hogeland, 1973). Nursing, like feminist theory until the mid-1980s, tended to attribute falsely to all women and all nurses the viewpoints of white middle-class women of Western European and North American background (Nicholson, 1990).

Nursing also tends to see only itself in the mirror. With the exception of an occasional nod to nursing's medieval military and religious derivations, its pedagogical history tends to acknowledge little prior to Florence Nightingale. Even the profound impact of the historical theme of democratization from the seventeenth century on, and of the Industrial Revolution with its resultant cataclysmic reorganization of life in Europe and North America, get relatively little attention—despite their overarching implications for redefining women's roles. Nursing comes directly from that unsettled period of transition between medieval and contemporary orientations. But even in its reification of Florence Nightingale's belief in the value of unceasing nursing care, nursing history seldom notes her powerful influence on development of hospitals and hospital administration (Nightingale, 1858, 1859a, 1859b). Nursing's pedagogies never exist alone, and thus cannot be fruitfully examined in isolation; the story must be historicized as a whole. The way an interpreter constructs meanings when representing that past portrays beliefs and behaviors that make sense in the present. The extent to which the reader can understand how past reality was experienced by those living at the time is always open to question. While the past cannot be changed, its meanings can be revisited and revised and its values and beliefs articulated as a collective symbolic world view that serves as a master narrative (Comaroff & Comaroff, 1992).

Built on the bringing together of ethnography (the written interpretation of a culture) and historiography (the study of written history), historical anthropology explores processes that make and transform a particular world, thus delving deeply into the "mute meanings" (Comaroff & Comaroff, 1992, p. 35) inherent in actual practices. Fair representing becomes a realizable goal as social constructions once held to be inevitable and natural are recognized as merely culturally persistent and politically arbitrary. This is where anthropology contributes uniquely in the unfolding of new understandings. Located between the social sciences and the humanities (Kleinman, 1995), it recognizes that, juxtaposed with the sheer complexity of society, it is the specific social provenance of what appears in the historical context that matters. Logically, the more diverse the voices to be represented, the more threatened is the traditional historical discursive construction (Berkhofer, 1995). In the big picture, isolated incidents are of relatively little interest. Historical understanding comes in reference to the unfolding relationship of the phenomenon in the wider context.

Although newer strategies of historiography help interpret pasts clouded by contemporary perceptions and refocus away from past biases, a tendency to analyze in linear fashion can insinuate itself as if a given line of ideology predominates at all levels of experience (Deloria, 1985). The history of nursing's pedagogies is one of the rationality inherently embedded in the languages of education, science, medicine, hospitals, industry, labor, and nursing itself. Although clearly proceeding from a historical and cultural context, rationality is often touted as value-free and neutral, which results in a stripping of context and history and acceptance of an ahistorical, objectified way of relating to the world (Hiraki, 1992). That pattern of thinking does little to account for the total configuration of any situation, let alone a comprehensive understanding of nursing's pedagogies over time. Critique of any master narrative involves uncovering the power relations embedded in the language, communications, and social relations of a tradition. Hegemony inserts itself into history in the form of mute constructs and conventional practices originating in the assertions of one group but coming to permeate a political community (Comaroff & Comaroff, 1992). When those relations by which power is distributed are made explicit, they become negotiable and threaten hegemony.

In recent decades, the study of history has become more interdisciplinary and overtly interpretive (Berkhofer, 1995). Late modern and postmodern historicism extends beyond concerns about the ability of modern language to represent that "actual past" for modern consumption. Although constructivist views of history are difficult to assess for accuracy in depiction of a past original, it is also recognized that the best that can be done with any past circumstances is always a modern recreation. Poststructuralist and multiculturalist theoretical quandaries about "Who can speak for whom in history?" attest to the folly of seeking universality of viewpoint and knowledge (Berkhofer, 1995, p. 3). Take feminism, which, as "a world-view that values women and confronts systematic injustices based on gender" (Chinn & Wheeler, 1985), may help broaden understanding but can also be used merely to substitute one view for another by underscoring the limited positions of women or by bleaching "women of color into a social invisibility" (Donaldson, 1992, p. 16). There is no universalist historiography or omniscient history-telling of gender, race, ethnicity, or any other social distinction, including occupational discipline. In sum, all history is parochial. However, because history is fundamentally more ideological than objective and factual, and ideologies rarely exist in the singular, it takes a cultural view of history to reveal the domains of contest inherent in society and the confrontation of power along its fault lines (Comaroff & Comaroff, 1992).

Creating a historical interpretation of nursing's pedagogies threatened to be both incomplete and unwieldy. It is clear that understanding the evolution of nursing education and its constituents requires the histories of persons, places, and times, as well as the exploration of multiple ideologies, hegemonic forces, and interactions among contested meanings. These complex realities precluded the existence of any single, fixed, and unified meaning of nursing's pedagogies' historical text. Instead, what was revealed involved multiple and conflicting stories and alternative histories, including some that are strongly class-based and gendered, generational, or otherwise stratified. Women function, to some extent, in a separate culture within the culture they share with men. Women's culture is in large part unrecorded and unrecognized (Lerner, 1997). However, in history, women should not be characterized with a "separate but equal" conceptual framework, for that perpetuates the notion of their inferiority and the appropriateness of their marginalization; they must be related to the climate of opinion within which they lived or live (Hogeland, 1973). Tracing those social productions amounts to demystifying societal relationships to reveal socially interactive groups and systematically patterned distributions of power that contextualize interrelated social phenomena (Berkhofer, 1995). That is, in large part, why history is important as memory and as a source of identity. But history is also about collective immortality, since it keeps the past alive and gives coherence to the making and sharing of ideas, values, and experiences that become cultural tradition (Lerner, 1997).

A historical-anthropological study begins by constructing its own archive with its texts anchored in the processes of their production and connection (Comaroff & Comaroff, 1992). It was there that I began this chapter. A year of reading the methods and approaches of history and the histories of science, medicine, professionalism, industry and labor, education, nursing, and women resulted in hundreds of pages of notes, which I repeatedly searched for patterns, themes, interrelationships, and signs of change. The emerging narratives provoked me to think, and my thinking wended its way toward new narrative. Nursing's stories are not simply about women, nurses, physicians, or bedpans, but about all of those and innumerable other constituents in the material and immaterial contexts (and crises) of their representation, legitimation, and praxis (Denzin, 1997). On the other hand, I soon realized that much that has been written has already been so overanalyzed that it was unable to relate reliable, meaningful, and contextualized answers to my broad question. Nursing's pedagogical history, in addition to reflecting the waxing and waning of a century of higher education, is interwoven with (and both into and out of) the emergence of the rest of that list of influences: education, science, medicine, hospitals, industry, and the health-care professions—all as they relate to women and women's issues. And each of those harkens back to earlier philosophical, ethical, and ideological derivations. In sum, revealing history means creatively giving form and making meaning out of amorphous masses of material (Lerner, 1997). For this study, that meant going back to many primary sources, in addition to others' analyses and interpretations.

My own hybrid background in nursing and anthropology has given me many reasons to try to understand better the interface of these seemingly disparate yet essentially parallel ways of knowing and bodies of knowledge. My anthropological dissertation on the adaptive strategies of nurses sensitized me long ago to the profound and insidious ramifications of power on, in, and through nurses and physicians. Nursing's histories and pedagogies, even viewed critically to illuminate issues of power, could not comfortably be reduced to traditional historical lineages. Trying to understand how nursing came to be what it is and how nurses came to be who they are meant revealing and recreating the intersections of not only nursing's story, but aspects of other stories. In such an analysis, there is no simple return to the data to verify the facts, for those were interpreted—hopefully in context yet unabashedly displaced in time and place. I periodically tested my interpretations on experienced nurses from every type of educational background and any social scientist I could press into reviewing the massing manuscript. Despite viewing the construction of this chapter as the production of narrative, I desired a three-dimensional image in lieu of the traditional two-dimensional paper model to embody my interpretation of the history of nursing pedagogies. To accommodate this want, I chose an imaginary mirror-lined sphere. In the sphere's many smaller mirrors and lenses, the specter of the recreated stories integral to nursing's pedagogies reflect on each other and become visible from many perspectives and in any juxtaposition. Today, nursing faces some critical choices. Its survival depends on putting new lenses in the mirror to foster looking outward and to allow the legacy of cultural hegemony to be seen and acknowledged. It is my hope that this chapter will help bring about that change, for my study left me convinced that gleaning the intricacies of nursing's hegemonic cultural legacy is crucial to the pedagogical transformation upon which the discipline's future rests.

Part 1: Pre-Pedagogical Mirrors and Origins

The Mirrors of Western Tradition and Ideology

Exploring the history of nursing requires a critical look at numerous patterns, interrelationships, and changes involving ideas and practices, some ideal and some real, but most of them deeply rooted. With the monotheism of Western tradition legitimating the idea of a single, underlying, universalizable truth (Kleinman, 1995), the roots of nursing's pedagogies are firmly embedded in the extraordinarily ingrained, hierarchically stratified, unitary Western paradigm that for centuries has viewed the universe as polarized in sets of opposing categories. Replete with moral connotations, this view of oppositional dualism allows the world to be assessed in no uncertain terms: peoples and their lifeways can be "civilized" or "primitive," "Christian" or "pagan," "public" or "private," "us" or "them," every phenomenon right or wrong, good or bad— never both (Césaire, 1972; Hernández, 1997; Tsosie, 2000). There is a single valid and preferred version of any entity and phenomenon.

Confounded with this monistic dichotomization of nearly every aspect of living is a linguistically ingrained cultural tendency to genderize. Thus the allegedly male domain of the public arena and market place is countered by its binary opposite—the private, domestic sphere of females. While the Puritan ethic accorded European women some prestige for being dutiful wives and mothers (that is, faithful, submissive, pious, and hardworking in relation to males), "bad" women were by definition their behavioral and hegemonic opposites (promiscuous, assertive, impious, and fatigable). The centrality of women in colonial American society did not prevent men's psychological objectification of women's "otherness" (Cott, 1972). The era's world view afforded little opportunity for complementary relationships or individual autonomy.

European American culture, increasingly commercial and less agricultural, boomed during the eighteenth and nineteenth centuries. Society reeled at and reveled in material and immaterial change: new factories, inventions, and means of transportation; new opportunities, risks, expectations, and rules. By the mid–nineteenth century, American women were less likely to be making cloth than purchasing it (Douglas, 1977). As railroads and steamships outsped horses and sailing vessels, the tempo of life rapidly and radically increased. The lament was similar to today's: Victorians thought their lives were being shaped by haste and innovation, often at the price of time for reflection. Even idleness was energized—adventuresome excursions, exciting new novels, and peeps through microscopes at the unimaginable (Canedy, 1979).

Into this fervor, Charles Darwin's *Origin of Species* and Florence Nightingale's *Notes on Nursing* were published in 1859. Although both works were of immediate import, responses to them had little in common other than their timing. Society has a tendency to act as if the function of women as mothers, and hence the caring associated with nurturance, were essential to group survival and to be protected against any change. In American history the male conventional wisdom reflected English law, and more decisively, Puritan Protestant religious tenets and covert discrimination against white women. (Discrimination against nonwhite women was decidedly more overt.) At the same time, men often engaged in paternalistic indulgence (Hogeland, 1973). Although the new, competitive economic market orientation extended only indirectly to women, social expectations of family-focused roles and statuses were no longer automatic (Ehrenreich & English, 1978). Whatever possibilities may have existed, the "woman question"—that is, what societal change really meant in terms of women's roles—was soon answered ideologically by nineteenth-century "domestic feminism."

Change in women's roles is unsettling and even anathema to those in positions of established privilege, who traditionally viewed women as the simple preservers of established values (Canedy, 1979). Promoting women's education within the sphere of domesticity (thus making future mothers and wives more capable while remaining nonthreatening adjuncts to men and families [Lewenson, 1996]), made sense and had appeal. This classic solution exemplifies the ideological legitimation of beliefs and values that are congenial with existing expectations. Naturalizing values and practices that only superficially challenge the status quo effectively excludes rival tracks of thought while making the acceptable choices seem self-evident and inevitable (Donaldson, 1992). Alexis de Tocqueville, famous for his analysis of democracy in America after his tour in 1831, noted that American women, like those of other Protestant nations, had more autonomy than women in Catholic countries. However, he also noted that care was taken in America to sustain two clearly distinct trajectories for the sexes to keep them in different albeit generally equitable paths, although the intellects of women were restrained by their schooling and methods of teaching, which served more to occupy time and produce companionship than to educate. Nineteenth-century American "ladies" were typically literary, so their minds were not vacuous. But readers were more plentiful than thinkers.

The Technical Working Mirror

Women have worked outside their homes for causes related to nursing at least since the times of medieval religious societies. They continued to do so until the sixteenth century, when the Protestant Reformation resulted in a sharp reduction in Northern Europe of the predominantly Catholic religious orders in hospitals (Glass & Brand, 1979). In agricultural America, families rather than individuals were the functioning productive unit in rural communities. The farm was both home and the place of work, with men's and women's tasks complementary parts of a whole. Domestic crafts were important and brought esteem. Nonagricultural, nondomestic occupations (such as trades, shopkeeping, and innkeeping) that were part of town life were also frequently carried on by families (Cott, 1972). Production roles changed and became gendered as industrialization advanced and shrunk women's opportunities in business and the retail trades. Gender differentiation gained momentum as industrialization did. By 1830 women ran primarily only those stores that exclusively served women (Hogeland, 1973). As nineteenth-century American men became less focused on creating a righteous society and more concerned with material acquisitions, they promoted an ideology that obligated women to personify goodness. It seemed that the more freedom men gained in public life, the more they wanted women's delicate "natures" restrained to the context of the home (Harris, 1978; Hogeland, 1973).

New technology that accompanied industrialization reduced menial household work for some women, primarily those who were white and who lived in towns. Running water eliminated parades of buckets. Electricity expanded the hours of light. Women bought more and canned, wove, and gardened less as they made the cultural transition from producers to consumers (Rothman, 1978). However, changing ideas about social prestige still prevented women from translating the extra time into employment outside the home. That was acceptable only for brief times before marriage or, to relieve the tedium presumed to fill the lives of unmarried women. With the crystallization of an American middle class that held economic and political prominence, people were no longer so much viewed as born into social roles and statuses, but rather as able to change those with effort and resources. Work was increasingly a means of climbing the social ladder. Women, by participating in social rather than in public life, provided an element of stability in the rapidly changing culture (Canedy, 1979).

Men learned to function independently in the industrializing society, while women's roles avoided any competition with the world of men. A "separate sphere" emerged in which middle-class women, as private and amateur figures, were expected to care for their homes while their husbands attended to business outside them (Lewenson, 1996; Margolis, 1984). Those women who worked outside the home typically taught, learned to type, or worked as shop clerks—although employers seldom hired women when men were willing or able to fill the positions. Prior to the interdependent developments of hospitals and modern nursing, few career opportunities existed beyond teaching, needlework, keeping boarders, household service, and being private governesses (Kalisch & Kalisch, 1995; Lewenson, 1996). If one had money and social prestige, the options might be somewhat greater, but women typically remained barred from public (that is, outside-the-home) positions (Canedy, 1979). Meanwhile, whatever their socioeconomic situations, women were generally expected to "embody and propagate an inherently feminine kind of morality, chastity, and sensibility" (Rothman, 1978, p. 5).

Concurrent with society's proliferation of new criteria for prestige and specifications for proper women's roles, a widening gap between rich and poor saw some people investing in the lucrative products of new technologies while others struggled to get by. Economic circumstances could shift quickly in nineteenth-century America, leaving women particularly vulnerable since their economic positions, like their social statuses, generally depended on their households. Yet employment outside the home invited chronic underemployment in service as governesses and lady companions, or, if one lacked social standing, factory or mill work (Canedy, 1979). Women's aspirations typically by-passed the marketplace in favor of the security of the home sphere and the middle-class ideal of domesticity (Ehrenreich & English, 1978).

Overall, the social position of American women declined between the colonial period and second half of the nineteenth century. Initially there was a shortage of women, and their economic function was valued, but this changed by 1840 as distinctions between the work of men and women in factories increased and women's work became more competi-tive, cheaper, and less skilled (Hogeland, 1973). Both men and women, on the other hand, expected men to out-earn women because men did more lucrative types of work (men were automatically preferred over women for advancement since women were—ideally—interested in serving others and society rather than in salaries). In addition to the rationalization of lesser salaries as adequate for women, women were expected to work only until they married (Flood, 1981).

To understand nursing in the United States, it is important to con-sider more global issues around women's roles and production than those pertinent only to postcolonial North American society. The situa-tion in the United States reflected the male bias that was and is the most common pattern in nation states. Only in far less technologically complex, traditional societies is equality between the sexes the norm (Etienne & Leacock, 1980). Women's roles are most valued by society when the dichotomy between the public and domestic spheres is least pronounced and women's contributions to subsistence are greatest (Kot-tak, 1999). Not only did social change wrought by industrialization result in the loss of privileges that many women had experienced, such as prac-tices of healing and midwifery (Cott, 1972), but nursing's pedagogical roots were institutionalized in the context of the "proper" place of women as secondary and deferential to men's more active roles. Some would argue that women were not absent from the workplace of male-dominated classical capitalism but merely present differently as service workers in feminized roles and members of "helping" occupations using mothering skills. But these were secondary roles, since women's full-time, primary, functions were as wives and mothers. The character of such arrangements only confirms the strong masculine bias of both capi-talist economics and the history of the industrial age (Fraser, 1987).

Certainly women's roles in the industrializing West included healing and caring for the sick. Women healers had virtually sole responsibility for childbirth and gynecological care throughout recorded history until the eighteenth century (Harding, 1980). In seventeenth-century healthcare, the idea of a man acting as a midwife was considered outrageous, but—with the contraction of acceptable roles for women and development of roles for male physicians—by the middle of the rapidly industrializing nineteenth century, the suggestion that women should train as physicians was equally shocking (Hogeland, 1973). Later, curing roles, which were seen as intellectual, manipulative, emotionally disengaged, and male, were separated from and were juxtaposed with caring roles, viewed as compassionate, nurturing, intuitive, and female. "Women are praised for assisting nature but not interfering with it" (Glass & Brand, 1979, p. 39). Overall, while traditional female activities were ignored, the culture's ideals increasingly included the developing professions and ways of life that rose above the exigencies of necessity. With the stuff of everyday life insignificant (Norris, 1998), the social convention that women were responsible for caring for sick and feeble family members profoundly affected female psychology and tied women closely to their homes (Lerner, 1977).

The Schooling Mirror

Changes in the organization of society led nineteenth-century formal education into costly gentility (Douglas, 1977). In the United States, for those who could afford them, women's colleges developed to account for the time young women no longer spent discharging domestic responsibilities (Rothman, 1978). For the most part, girls' education generally remained rooted in the home, while the societal resources (that is, prestige, power, and wealth) that shaped the roles of married women were acquired through males. Hence, although socially significant accomplishments were to be useful in society, women rarely had opportunities to achieve beyond the domestic realm. Florence Nightingale, who refused to submerge her intellectual side, wrote in 1850 that she saw herself as having three choices: being a literary woman (which generally meant reading and writing at home), a married woman, or a hospital sister (Woodham-Smith, 1951). Her mother and her sister exemplified society's expectations of women. It is hypothesized that the stress Nightingale experienced as a result of the conflict between her choices and Victorian society's expectations was among the reasons she took to her bed for much of her life (Canedy, 1979).

When public schools were founded in the 1820s, it was assumed that educated, sober, and refined young men would teach in them. In reality, many teachers were poorly educated or taught only long enough to become established in some other field. State normal schools developed to prepare teachers and attracted women—whom many thought naturally better fitted than men to the role by temperament, habit, and circumstances. Although the turnover was high, women worked for low pay and were generally pliable, given the absence of competing opportunities. In a wage economy, the lower paying an occupation is, the more likely it is to be equally staffed by men and women or to be predominantly female (Lerner, 1997). Teaching was no exception. Class differences in the United States, firmly established as gendered, carried over into schooling; age was less an issue. As educational systems grew, women taught younger children and they taught about women's work—such as home care and nursing.

Ideologically, public schooling exemplified the use of a singular world view to support the traditional dichotomies with inauthentic equations. In many minds and policies, education was as closely associated with cultural assimilation as Christianity was linked conceptually to civilization. These monistic associations supported colonialist and racist consequences (Donaldson, 1992). At the same time, since women were primed to be responsible for the moral upbringing of children, mothering was held to be synonymous with teaching. Such was the role of the "pioneer mothers of the republic," who were grandly credited with shaping and guiding society (Fowler, 1886). Teaching, meanwhile, being numerically "feminized" in its quasi-public sector, settled precariously into a status that was neither part of the state bureaucracy nor part of the individualist market of private industry (Blackmore, 2000). Instead, teaching was taken for granted, like other activities such as mothering, as basic to the survival of the species (Nicholson, 1987). Later, this dialectic put occupational nursing into a limbo similar to teaching's and transferred the same profound implications of ambiguity to nursing's pedagogies.

The Socioreligious Familial Mirror

Between 1820 and 1875, America's strict Calvinist Protestantism lost much of its rigidity and the country metamorphosed into the world's most powerfully aggressive capitalistic system. Adam Smith, an influential eighteenth-century philosopher, had broken important theoretical ground by asserting that the common good was best met by everyone acting in his or her own interests. With this ideology empowering the free market (Greenleaf, 1988), new approaches to communication and scientific knowledge blossomed. Any skepticism about science and its authority fell to the rationalization revealed in new discoveries. It was all somewhat daunting and confusing, but doubt consistently fell short of "denial of the mind as a valid instrument of truth" (Canedy, 1979, p. 8). Nonetheless, mainstream society lost confidence in its ability to perceive the "ultimate" truths thought to be inherent in religion, ethics, and aesthetics.

Gender is sometimes viewed as a status group involving real or potential oppression analogous to race or class. At other times, women's issues are thought to differ significantly from those of groups framed by race or class (because women's responses tend to differ from those of other groups when oppressed) and simply to reflect variable situations of interdependence (Whyte, 1978). It is sometimes mistakenly assumed that the subordination of women is or has been culturally universal. There are phenomena, such as pregnancy, lactation, and early childcare, that characterize women everywhere, but there is no worldwide social position for women. Historically in the United States, women's circumstances remained linked directly to those of children throughout shifts in expectations of "woman's proper place." In a society in which the idealized prototype was an enterprising young man on the make, the desirable role for women was to enhance (emphasizing decorous conduct and matters of taste, delicacy, innocence, and sentiment) rather than sustain (Cott, 1972). The ideal of true womanhood and its corollary cult of domesticity remained the normative behavior toward which women were expected to, and usually did, strive. For many of those who could afford it, the nineteenth-century replacement for women's earlier role in family productivity was one of idleness expressed positively as gentility, decorative worth, and beauty predicated upon frailty, purity, and asexuality (Gordon & Buhle, 1976; Welter, 1966).

True womanhood held four cardinal virtues: piety, purity, submissiveness, and domesticity, which translated readily into mother, daughter, sister, and wife (Hogeland, 1973). Cultural manifestations of idealized "true womanhood" were religion-like in their strict ritual and dogmas, including new demands expressed in a subtle but significant language of repression. During this time, leg became "limb," the breast of the chicken became "light meat," women were referred to as "ladies" or "females," and pregnancy involved increasing secrecy or, if necessary, "being with child" or "woman's condition" (Gordon & Buhle, 1976). Women's morally superior nature depended on the absence of sexual participation, which was generally stereotyped as painful and humiliating, save for the satisfaction of husbands and the propagation of the species. Relationships between husband and wife were in large part based upon property. Promiscuity was permissible only for men, a situation that supported prostitution, for which an unmarried woman who was no longer a virgin (and was therefore "ruined") was conveniently suited.

The principles and consequences of U.S. social policy toward women present an intricate history of women's place in society. Yet conflicting efforts to promote the welfare of women did little to alter their situation because of the assumption that change would have a negative impact on the welfare of children or the integrity of the family. As mothers, women were to instill obedience in their young early on. After the Civil War, expectations mellowed somewhat: children were to be raised with love and affection, their vitality guided with sympathy and interest, but their wills were not to be broken and their punishment was not to be corporeal (Rothman, 1978). Evidence abounded that it was unwise to raise daughters as if marriage were the only possibility of a livelihood, yet marriage and manners were the foremost expectations of women. Despite their presumed fragility, impracticality, emotionality, and instability, womanhood on its pedestal was to uphold virtue and guard the culture, in addition to (out of sheer necessity) propagating the species and restraining the unruly instincts of men (Kalisch & Kalisch, 1995; Rothman, 1978).

Cultural change was rapid and wide-ranging. In the eighteenth century, life grew gradually more secularized and materialistic. Guidelines and attitudes were generally European with women's "proper" duties strongly influenced by transatlantic colonial cultures. Even in the nineteenth century, woman's status and role in the family and in God's plan, according to the prevailing Christian ideology, remained the primary and often the only sources of power for women (Cott, 1972). In addition to tending families, self-sacrificing women involved themselves with charities and reform efforts. It was a time of fervent, evangelizing colonialism. A feminine fusion of clerical and pedagogical roles merged in the conviction that ministers could do little without the aid of self-denying female teachers (Rothman, 1978). Thousands of American women contributed large sums and much of their lives to missionary efforts. While housewives strove to form the minds of their children, feminine missionaries endeavored to save "souls from terrible ignorance" (Douglas, 1977, p. 106). Vindicating themselves through feminine self-sacrifice, many women came as close as they ever would to jobs like those men held through their participation in religious activity (Cott, 1972; Giele, 1995). Religion helped women resolve the conflict between their heavy responsibilities and their lack of power by defining their identities, countering their isolation and shaping their connections to their communities.

The nineteenth-century family, with its rituals and social life, was more central to individual experience than during the previous century, when men more often sought the company of other men. The home took on an almost fetishistic need to be cultivated internally, rather than in terms of community function (Cott, 1972). Now home life was valued as a refuge from politics and economics, and from the social world with its strict etiquette and rules for acceptance and rejection. At the same time, however, expanding geographical mobility increasingly stretched old expectations about relationships with family and kin (Canedy, 1979). Virtuous motherhood demanded both creativity and a core of fixed rigidity as, with each decade, an increasing number of women moved from rural areas to confront living in increasingly diverse urban environments. Industrialization affected nearly all ways of life. By the middle of the nineteenth century, while the majority of America's population still lived on the land despite rapid growth of the cities, and more than 95% of women remained at home as their mothers had before them, traditional home crafts were disappearing into factory production (Ehrenreich & English, 1978). Clergy, popular magazines, and politicians harped on the home and home life as sacred and endangered as hundreds of thousands of immigrants poured into the "land of opportunity." While American ethnic diversity burgeoned, society drew stark lines of race and class.

The Healing Mirror

Colonial America had few defenses against disease and sickness. Eventually, society developed almshouses for the poor and pesthouses for the contagious, but there were no real hospitals. Female healers treated the sick on the basis of experience, while male healers more often worked through faith or resorted to heroic measures such as massive bleeding, potent laxatives, or emetics (Glass & Brand, 1979; Kalisch & Kalisch, 1995). Still a century away from the medicalization that characterized twentieth-century America, the 1830s saw the Popular Health Movement, in which converged a "workingman's movement" and a woman's movement, rendering health and feminist concerns essentially indistinguishable (Baxandall, Gordon & Reverby, 1976; Ehrenreich & English, 1978).

Medical work was not well thought of in the eighteenth and nineteenth centuries. Even after 1800, when medical schools on the east coast began producing a trickle of trained physicians and surgeons to replace poorly prepared, apprenticed practitioners, the United States trailed far behind Europe in healthcare. Until the Civil War in the 1860s, medical standards generally declined as the population grew (Kaufman, 1976). Medical intervention often did more to aggravate than alleviate disease with whiskey, herbs, heavy metals, and fomentations as the treatments of choice (Kalisch & Kalisch, 1995). Yet, in less than a century, curative biomedicine emerged from being a cottage industry into a highly complex division of labor surrounded by huge industries and at the height of public prestige, power, and authority (Coburn & Willis, 2000; Joralemon, 1999). Biomedicine pressed the practitioner to recognize patterns of disordered biological processes and diagnostic categories. There was little place in that narrow disease-focused therapeutic vision for the patient's experience of suffering (Kleinman, 1995) or for the need for care in addition to treatment.

While it is often assumed that medicine gained its authority through an increasing ability to improve health or prevent or cure disease, social scientists and historians conclude that medicine rose to power before it was truly efficacious and that improvements in health conditions were shaped more by changes in social and environmental conditions than by medical expertise (Brown, 1998; Coburn & Willis, 2000; Conrad & Kern, 1994; Good, 1998). To understand the historical development of medicine in the United States, one must place it in the context of a larger movement of the rise of professions. As a profession, medicine is rooted in the guilds of the Middle Ages. Changes in society encouraged medical professionals to increase their social position and power by using professional exclusionary strategies to gain and maintain a market monopoly. The time was right for biomedicine to prosper as a profession. Social, political, and economic factors (such as the appeal of science and the dominance of curative over preventive medicine) fit hand-in-glove with the interests and ideology of a rising class of industrialists (Coburn & Willis, 2000; Navarro, 1976). The medical profession, motivated in large part by profit and driven by rationality and efficiency, learned quickly how to control its own education, numbers, and activities (Kaufman, 1976). Scientific medicine was congruent with scientific management in industry and in education, while medicine's individualist and mechanistic orientation obscured the social causes of disease. Carefully controlling knowledge and its use, physicians were soon labeled public authorities on all things having to do with health. In an age of monopolies, medicine became an exemplar.

Curative medicine has long been accused of serving as a vehicle for the production and reproduction of traditional paternalistic modes of control (Ehrenreich & English, 1978; Joralemon, 1999). Radical feminist views of medical history emphasize that the medical profession has usurped formerly female-dominated health-related activities, subordinated women, excluded women from active healing roles and driven women into health auxiliary groups charged with the "uniquely feminine" roles of caring and housekeeping (Coburn & Willis, 2000). Indeed, in the paradigm of professional authority, women in North America were deprived of their roles in healing and saw their communal bonds weakened—bonds based on skill and women sharing information among themselves. Medical training shifted from apprenticeships and classical training in Greek and the humanities to a university-based education in science and in biology especially—which fit well with the need to control infectious and acute disease and allowed clinical autonomy to rest in the hands of a highly technically prepared few. The "regular" doctor (in contrast to a mélange of popular "irregular" eclectics, botanists, homeopaths, herbalists, hydropaths, and others, in addition to women practicing traditional healing ways) set out to compete with disease and to disarm it (Ehrenreich & English, 1978).

The female caring occupations—and their newly developing pedagogies—became part of modern healthcare at a time when it was widely accepted that women's roles in the public sphere should not be technical, but could, should, and would parallel those they filled in the home. The evolving healthcare system reflected the gender biases and dichotomies that underlay the Western tradition. In the realm of healing, that meant that men were readily viewed as developing expertise through systematic training and formal mechanisms of accountability, while women gained knowledge through experience. With the insistent reification of scientific thinking at all levels of society, the experiential knowing of women was increasingly considered outside of science and therefore inconsequential. Women, whether nurses, midwives, ritual specialists, or simply maternal carriers of culture, were seen traditionally as informal healers whose healing roles were first and foremost part of the mother metaphor (Apple, 1992; McClain, 1989).

The Scientific Mirror

There seemed no limit to the potential inherent in the rise of science. More than a transformative force that could elevate medicine above its commercial competitors, the age of science coincided with a period of frenzied industrialization from about 1840 on. Providing a shared culture for innovators of the nineteenth century, scientism was viewed as good and moral, and as a source of almost neoreligious reform. This was an era of rapid change and developing professionalism, while humanitarianism was deemed sentimental and hazardous to progress. Social work, which was a voluntary activity before the 1880s, used science to professionalize itself. Even housekeeping and child raising became "scientific" (Ehrenreich & English, 1978; Lobove, 1965), as did nursing and teaching.

Ideologically, it was assumed that everyone had an assigned place in the scientific order of things. With nineteenth-century scientists blithely applying the results of biological studies to human society, any attempt to abdicate one's place in the natural order was construed as inappropriate to the point of being pathological. Darwin's theory of evolution so neatly fit explanations of the sexes and human races as different evolutionary phenomena that a "verifying" body of evidence was soon produced. By the 1860s, women and African Americans came in last in the United States' social ordering, both being viewed as too primitive to be innovators, experts, or specialists. The question no longer was what women could do, but what they ought to do. By 1900, with big money available to support elite professions and universities, social Darwinism prevailed. Wealth generated through industrialization made the university system possible, and only now, at the start of the twenty-first century, is globalization of the political economy destabilizing patterns of university professional work developed over the past century (Slaughter & Leslie, 1997; Morrow & Torres, 2000). In the arena of health, while much "medical" knowledge has been developed by nonphysicians, it has been developed within hospitals, medical schools and medical centers administratively controlled by physicians (Coburn & Willis, 2000). In sum, with the nineteenth-century emergence of the modern university and the professions, physicians were able to control the organization of healthcare as well as medicine, while they resisted corporate domination by making use of the skills of nurses and others (Flood, 1981; Greenleaf, 1988; Harding, 1980).

The Domestic Mirror

In the heyday of professionalization and reform, domestic science became a way of life. Expertise based on systematizing information on housekeeping was made available to such large numbers of women that by 1900 hundreds of teachers and social workers saw themselves as experts on homemaking. Science had answered "the woman question." What does a woman do with her life? She lives a scientific domestic life referred to as "right living." In response to increasing industrialization and urbanization, indoctrination aimed at enhancing and preserving health and home life began in elementary school. "Domestic science" built on that in secondary school, home economics in the normal and professional (that is, technical) schools, and "euthenics" in colleges and universities (Ehrenreich & English, 1978). Although by 1900 infant mortality was decreasing due to improvements in nutrition and sanitation, medical practitioners held that domestic science was the answer to infant mortality, contagious disease, intemperate use of food and drink, divorce, insanity, pauperism, and competition between the sexes (Ehrenreich & English, 1978; "Public school information on cooking," 1899). Kitchen skills were transformed into laboratory exercises, and budgeting reframed as economics. The Germ Theory shaped cleaning and inculcated a severe and persevering public anxiety about contagion.

Given the dread and history of high infant mortality, mothers listened to any admonition associated with combating disease. Reformers aimed for a totality of "right living" in single-family, owner-occupied American homes with explicit expectations for every aspect of life, including the moral and spiritual. A lack of scientific evidence to support a correlation between thorough house cleaning and family health did not undermine the romantic commitment to "home values" and the equation of cleanliness with not only godliness, but Americanism itself—while nutrition ethnocentrically represented middle-class appetites. By the 1920s, proliferating high school "household arts" courses supposedly introduced ideas leading to "higher ideals" and culture (Ehrenreich & English, 1978). The stage was set for cultural dependence on technology and behaviorism.

The Feminine, Feminist, and Hegemonic Mirror

American interpretations of sex, race, and class seem inevitably to involve power and therefore must be explored in those terms. Male domination cannot be presumed to be universal, but European colonialism has often made it appear that way. Consider the power-induced asymmetry that resulted in the Americas when European colonization there denigrated the autonomy of indigenous women who traditionally experienced more egalitarian relationships than either European or European American women did. From colonial times through the Victorian era, Americans viewed women in non-Western societies as oppressed, servile, and subject to being liberated by "progress" and "civilization" (Etienne & Leacock, 1980). Capitalism ascended in Europe through the process of colonial exploitation, linking the general subjugation of whole peoples with the subjugation of women. Combining political prowess with a ubiquitous colonial divide-and-rule strategy (by which Christian churches sought to impose a model of the patriarchal European nuclear family), Europeanized norms for domestic and conjugal behavior became the only standards considered "proper" and "civilized" (Donaldson, 1992; Etienne & Leacock, 1980).

Women responded to finding themselves segregated from men by affiliating themselves with extra-familial groups. Many of those were women's clubs, reform associations, and philanthropic societies set on making "all women over in the image of virtuous motherhood" (Rothman, 1978, p. 5). In the United States before the Civil War, abolitionist and women's-rights movements shared both ideals and supporters, just as concern for workmen's health and women's issues had earlier. Benevolent associations, charitable institutions, and mutual support groups provided settings for the support of the antislavery abolition movement and later the women's suffrage movement (Ehrenreich & English, 1978). Abolitionist concerns led eventually to the organization of the women's rights movement in the United States, the overall cause being "the school of *human* rights" (emphasis in the original) (Grimké, 1838, p. 126). That first generation of American feminists, those members of the "woman movement" such as Lucretia Mott and Elizabeth Cady Stanton who declared their belief in equality of men and women in writing by the 1840s, were pragmatic in their reasoning. Women had less support than slaves, for whose freedom abolitionists were actively campaigning. No matter how educated women might be, they had fewer rights than illiterate men who could vote. Efforts to gain rights for women began to gain momentum (Glass & Brand, 1979).

For all of that, American culture seemed intent on celebrating a perpetual Mother's Day. Replete with feminine purity, religious conformity, and redeeming activity, middle-class Protestant nineteenth-century American women sought to gain power through the exploitation of feminine identity as their society defined it (Douglas, 1977). This era constructed a blatantly artificial image of women with tiny waists and great hooped skirts that impeded movement—the antithesis of the way the era idealized ruggedly natural, adventurous, rapidly progressing men. Even into the twentieth century, there remained a romantic nostalgia of women as childlike innocents, much like stereotypes of indigenous peoples. Both were expected to be naturally amiable, tender and submissive, peaceful among themselves, affectionate, light-hearted and good-natured, oriented toward emotion and impulse, and outside the domain of sound quantitative reasoning (Ehrenreich & English, 1978).

Anatomy dictated destiny in Victorian America, and biology was destiny indeed since Victorian America lacked both safe and effective contraceptives and a sophisticated understanding of female reproductive processes. The professionalization of American medicine excluded women from medical schools while retaining an image of woman's body as that of a "natural invalid" (Cott, 1972, p. 20). Menstruation was viewed as a nervous susceptibility that could lead to full-blown hysteria, or at the very least, periodic infirmity. Physicians insisted that women's biology limited them to specific activities and female maladies that made active participation in the world outside the home unwise. Women were judged biologically, physically, and emotionally impaired, and were thought to be endangered by strenuous activity (Vertinsky, 1994). Nervous forces had to be protected, mental excitement avoided, physical and intellectual exercise curtailed, pregnancy and other functions viewed as disease, and tonics (often described as vegetable in nature but composed of opiates or laced with alcohol) employed to shore up fragile femininity (Rothman, 1978). Women did not own businesses or hold office, yet they were increasingly exempt from responsibilities of domestic industry. Those who did not have to work wrote or became aggressive about holy causes while men patronized them with moral oversight. Many women believed they were meant to take part in a mission to redeem society. The ethos intensified sentimentalism that both undermined the more intellectual values of Calvinistic culture and reinforced male hegemony in different guises (Douglas, 1977).

The place in history of the earlier "woman movement" was in large part obscured by later romantics who were less interested in rights than in guardianship and motherhood. The delicate, affluent lady who was completely dependent on her husband became the ideal of femininity for women of all classes (Ehrenreich & English, 1978). In the late nineteenth century, broader education in the humanities was overthrown and instruction in painting, music, and embroidery deemed sufficient for women (Kalisch & Kalisch, 1995)—which further limited their sphere of expression and influence. The ideal of being more civilized and moral than men, but sickly, frail and subject to mental and physical derangement, served to underline the common wisdom that women had best stay home. However, the repression of women's capacities for purposes of private property did not occur without a backlash. The curricula of reactionary women's colleges developing at the time included physical fitness programs along with other efforts toward equitable education, and physical exercise became the favorite remedy of the few women doctors in practice (Rothman, 1978).

In the nineteenth century, sexual repressiveness and ignorance about women's bodies precluded frank discussion of behavior, anatomy, physiology. Woman was defined by the reproductive aspects of her sex while expected to be sexless, except insofar as she tolerated the sexual content of marriage as a necessary accommodation in the cult of true womanhood (Cott, 1972; Welter, 1966). Overall, this was also an age of expertise by others in women's lives. Perhaps most telling about the position of women was the history of midwifery in the United States. Midwives had the monopoly on birthing from antiquity through colonial times. As late as 1910, they still attended at least half the births occurring in the United States (Litoff, 1992). Most midwives—particularly those who were apprentice-trained or untrained "neighbor women"—took a relatively noninterventionist approach, providing support and encouragement while nature took its course (Litoff, 1992). Given evidence that infant and maternal mortality rates for deliveries supervised by midwives were equal to or lower than those for deliveries supervised by most general practice physicians (Devitt, 1979), logically this approach to childbirth called for the establishment of midwifery programs similar to those already present in Europe. Instead however, between 1900 and 1930 in the United States, midwives were nearly totally eliminated, being either outlawed by the state or, more often, harassed into submission by local medical authorities. As the utility of obstetrics in building physi- cians' practices became apparent, female assistance at birth was increasingly defined as dangerous, improper, or even criminal—except where large immigrant or minority populations continued to press "ethnic specialists" into service (Dawley, 2000; Ehrenreich & English, 1978; Litoff, 1992). Many nurses joined physicians in the effort to abolish midwifery in favor of medical intervention, not realizing the profound ramifications their actions had for both nursing specialties and for women. Midwives, many of whom were isolated from each other by poverty, geography, and language barriers, lacked the resources needed to stand up to their critics (Litoff, 1992). With the elimination of midwifery, women generally fell under the biological hegemony of the medical profession. No longer autonomous healers, they could be only employees or customers.

Submission to hegemonic forces involves exchanges that are oppressive and result in psychological and social damage (Bulhan, 1985; Fanon, 1967). The oppression of women is often viewed as complicit in oppressive ideologies of race and class (Donaldson, 1992; Jackson, 1993), yet the histories of women and nursing and its pedagogies cannot be simplified to a picture of man as the colonizer and woman as the colonized. Each can be both, in what Freire (1970) referred to as "the reduction of the Other to the Same" (p. 140). Nurse training schools emerged (as becomes apparent upon examining the historical context) soon thereafter through a commercial orientation that helped advance the professional, psychological, and economic oppression of women through apprenticeship. Historically, the apprenticeship model served well as a means of keeping groups in subordinate positions and was used as an intermediary stage between servitude and freedom (Ashley, 1976). Remnants of apprenticeship pedagogies still haunt nursing and nursing education.

The Reforming, Progressive Mirror

Relatively little attention has been paid to the implications of rationalization for women workers and the development of the service industries, but the time during which modern nursing developed was
one in which women actively intervened to shape society (Melosh,
1982). It is not surprising that women organized nursing, just as they
did charity, reform, and social work. They transformed domestic function into public service, creating institutions and occupations in the
process. After the Civil War, women in the United States organized
themselves to promote the best interests of virtuous womanhood and
to set clear guidelines for the benevolent-minded. Alcohol, like contra-
ception, was to be banned; societies such as the Women's Christian
Temperance Union flourished. The settlement movement—attracting
gifted women and men and turning, as Jane Addams put it, a generation
of young Americans into reformers (Flexner, 1975)—sought to build a
new social order with community spirit and social cohesion in the turbu-
lent neighborhoods of recently arrived immigrants. Since social problems were seen as moral problems, solutions demanded the support of
philanthropy, reform, and social policy. A spirit of rectification was in
the air, although the ideology, class-bound and narrowly defined as it
was, focused on changing the person rather than the system (Rothman,
1978).

Meanwhile, the increasing influence of the professions, particularly
medicine, invaded women's sense of self. Those who thought such issues
mattered fought for access to professional education, birth control, sexual counseling, and preventive healthcare (Rothman, 1978). By the early
twentieth century, women took on new roles influenced by technological
and commercial growth. A meaningful few managed to become factory
inspectors, trade unionists, or journalists, or otherwise overreached the
curricula of the romantic era, but those exceptions were relatively rare.
At the same time, there were notable struggles with racism and other
divisions within the women's groups, so that many groups worked sepa-
rately along racially divided lines. Yet by 1900—when the *American
Journal of Nursing* was first published—the public was most concerned
about yellow fever, striking coal miners, the Boxer rebellion affecting
American missionaries in China, and virtually nothing directly to do with
women (Roberts, 1954).

Until the 1870s, nursing in the United States remained in the hands of the uneducated, with the exception of a few religious orders. Although some ten thousand women (and not a few men) served as nurses in the Civil War, there was no system or organization coordinating that effort. Women might be volunteer or paid; educated or uneducated; active participants or gawking observers; wives or sisters of soldiers, or unrelated to the servicemen; aristocratic or poor—but all were untrained and lacked clear duties, and medical personnel typically did not want them there (Kalisch & Kalisch, 1995; Roberts, 1954).

But military carnage did not present the only circumstances in which women developed active roles. Colonial America was a preindustrial society primarily British in its customs, but also affected by its advancement on a wilderness (Cott, 1972). As the American frontier pushed westward, women were always present on its fringes, active in publishing and other occupations such as medicine and law. They faced many of the same obstacles that women in the Eastern United States faced, but sometimes had more success in establishing themselves due to the need for their work. Midwifery and nursing were common occupations, although they seldom involved formal training or monetary remuneration, and they did not rate acknowledgment as gainful employment in the census or other official documents (Myers, 1982).

Part 2: The Mirrors of Nursing's Pedagogies

The Blessing Mirror

Prior to the twentieth century, hospitals were primarily repositories for the destitute and dying. One exception was at Kaiserwerth, Germany, at which attempts were made to improve care with the 1836 establishment of a school for training nurses. Nurses' training there resonated with the repression of monastic ideals of self-abnegation, strict obedience to authority, and dedication to duty (Glass & Brand, 1979). In 1860, Florence Nightingale, after having been to Kaiserwerth and applying what she learned there during the Crimean War, opened her nurse training school at St. Thomas Hospital in London (Roberts, 1937). The training of nurses fit well with the reform movements popular at the time (Glass & Brand, 1979). However, change again had conceptual and practical limits. Nightingale not only defined nursing as women's work but, while aware of the powerlessness of women, she set up a subservient relationship between nurses and physicians by ordering nurses to care for <u>only those pati</u>ents whom the doctors ordered them to see (Bush & Kjervik, 1979).

Meanwhile in the United States, society held that better educated women became better wives, mothers, and teachers. But teaching and saving souls did not prepare women to serve as nurses at home or on battlefields. The Crimean and American Civil wars revealed the need for sanitary conditions and, thus, organized nursing. At its 1868 meeting, the American Medical Association (<u>AMA) advocated training nurses</u> to upgrade nursing care in the United States to the level present in Europe. It was proposed that schools of nursing be formed under the aegis of county medical societies and attached to hospitals so that resident physicians and medical staff could provide instruction (Kalisch & Kalisch, 1995). Prior to the 1870s, women learned nursing through domestic practice and few received payment for the care they provided. Any woman could be called a nurse—from spinster relatives to the drunken prototypes characterized by Dickens's slovenly Sairey Gamp. The replacement of the "natural-born nurse" by trained nurses via formalized <u>apprenticeship training</u> challenged the limited role of domesticity in preparing women for their role in healthcare while it generally improved conditions in hospitals and demonstrated that nursing education had practical value. It also moved women beyond domesticity into public view (Lewenson, 1996). But the transition remained lodged in the foregone determination that women did nurturing and maintenance tasks while men dealt with the larger administrative and public aspects of the world (Flood, 1981; Harris, 1978).

Nursing and the Sanitary Hospital Mirror

In the mid–nineteenth century, hospitals in the United States were thought of as providing the barest custodial accommodation of strangers and the sick poor. Physical care in them was of little concern and typically construed as distasteful drudgery. General hospitals for all types of illnesses and all types of patients were rare, although medical practice was shifting—as techniques of antisepsis and asepsis became widely known and used—from patients' homes to hospitals that specialized in specific diseases (Melosh, 1982). Following upon advances in science, new medical, surgical, and laboratory resources conspired with tendencies toward smaller dwellings and a growing reliance among the general public on agencies outside the home to induce more patients to seek treatment in hospitals (Commission on Hospital Care, 1947; Vogel, 1980). Hospitals typically provided the basics: shelter, food, minimal assistance with activities of daily living, and physicians' treatments (Flood, 1981). Nightingale's sanitary reforms provided pure air, proper ventilation, nutritious food, and improved sanitary conditions in homes and hospitals alike. Her insistence that nurses undergo training programs transformed hospitals into safer environments than most homes were (Ashley, 1976; Lewenson, 1996). Keeping pace with Victorian-era expectations, the hospital's pupil nurses routinely cared for and kept meticulous notes on large numbers of patients (50 or more), swept and mopped floors, and dusted furniture and windowsills. The term "pupil" emphasized both the inferior status of the bearer and her submission to the control and responsibility of the institution (Flood, 1981). Duty was paramount; time off rare. Comportment was integral to an individual nurse's ability to project her worth and integrity (Aroskar, 1980).

Early hospitals usually specialized in specific diseases, such as tuberculosis (Connolly, 2000), but they soon reorganized under broader categories such as maternity, orthopedic, isolation, chronic, convalescent, or mental facilities (Kalisch & Kalisch, 1995; Roberts, 1954). Hospital insurance plans began around 1880. From early on, Blue Cross was the most popular. Blue Shield later added medical insurance (Kalisch & Kalisch, 1995). With federal funding, expanding third-party insurance, and overall public approval, hospitals proliferated as a prestigious and profitable service industry. Surgery, as the dominant intervention, became even more alluring to the public and medical practitioners with the techniques and knowledge developed during World War I (Hiestand, 2000; Roberts, 1954). Scientific industrial management central- ized many services, reducing the autonomy of the nurses on each floor (Melosh, 1982). The overall theme was rational efficiency through standardization and uniformity. Further revenue was produced from the sale of nursing services through registries for private duty nursing in homes, as well as in hospitals (Ashley, 1976). By the turn of the century, two or three new hospitals opened somewhere in the country every week, usually at the impetus of physicians who opposed development of public facilities. Municipalities built them rapidly and at times with little foresight (Commission on Hospital Care, 1947). As both the numbers of hospitals and numbers of larger (100 or more beds) hospitals increased, the question of who should control these business enterprises

loomed (Ashley, 1976; Vogel, 1980). While physicians made the executive decisions and determined hospital policies, most had medical practices outside the hospital and used the latter only for specific medical
endeavors, such as performing surgeries. They were not responsible for
the actual operating of the institutions (Ashley, 1976). Over time non-
medical and nonnursing personnel assumed administration of many of
the larger hospitals (Melosh, 1982).

Nursing played an integral part in the escalation in the number and
size of hospitals. When the first nursing schools in the United States
were opened in 1873, there were fewer than 200 hospitals in the entire
nation; by 1930 there were 7,416 (Melosh, 1982). The industry required
a disciplined workforce, so administrators attracted fee-paying clientele
by replacing untrained attendants with respectable pupil nurses. It became a circular phenomenon: better nursing brought in more fee-paying
patients. In 1910, one in four hospitals had a nursing school; by 1927,
several thousand hospitals kept their wards supplied with pupil nurses
(Melosh, 1982).

The Curricular Mirror

By 1890, 35 nurse training schools had been established with relatively high standards, given that 32% of their students had high school
educations, compared with only 2% of young women in the total population (Melosh, 1982). However, the uncontrolled proliferation of schools
downgraded overall admission standards to the extent that, in 1918, the
American Nurses Association (ANA) recommended that at least one
year of high school be successfully completed before entering nurse
training (Roberts, 1954). The age of admission had also dropped significantly (Flood, 1981). Arguments ensued about whether nurses were to
be trained in mechanical tasks or educated to think. Nursing struggled
with paternalistic ideology that sought to control its education and practice while promoting the notion that any woman, with minimal training,
could be a nurse. The literature echoes the widely held opinion that "A
nurse may be over-educated; she can never be over-trained" (Ashley,
1976, p. 77; Dorland, 1908). The type and quality of nursing education
was so scrutinized that it (rather than conditions of practice) became
the primary focus of early nurse leadership (Glass & Brand, 1979).

Hospital-centered training programs varied from those providing
simplified in-service patient care to those providing training and educa-

tional perspectives. Interestingly, the former "school-service" programs were most typical of university hospitals (Flood, 1981). By 1925, however, the fact that a high school education was not a prerequisite for entrance to nursing school provoked widespread concern about the quality of preparation. In addition to the limitations imposed by low admission standards, some schools had too few students to justify teaching staff to provide adequate instruction, while the learning value of the ward work depended on hospital size and the types of medical conditions encountered by student nurses (Kalisch & Kalisch, 1995; Melosh, 1982). Since loyalty to the hospital that housed the training program was highly valued by the hospital staff and administration, few training schools rotated students through different types of clinical services or sent them to other institutions. Students merely worked where they were most needed and learned what they could there. The only constant in hospital-based nurse training programs prior to the 1940s was the conflict they perpetuated between the goals of nursing education and those of medical institutions. Most schools had full time nursing faculty by the 1930s, but expectations focused on practical training rather than education and students continued to provide most of the nursing service in hospitals until well into the 1950s (Melosh, 1982).

Nurse training in the United States went through a pioneer period with a sketchy curriculum that was casually administered, and then boomed until 1913 along with public education. With curricula historically viewed as more of a guide than a standard, nursing curriculum development reflected an "orgy of overexpansion" of nurse training programs (Committee on Curriculum of the National League of Nursing Education, 1937). A lack of standards in training was exacerbated by the medical demands of World War I and the post-war influenza pandemic. New laws protected against the worst abuses, but wide variation in training continued. Overall, the period between 1913 and 1933 was at best one of stock-taking in nursing education policy. Amidst the dizzy inflation in numbers of schools and students, the first National League of Nursing Education (NLNE) curriculum was published in 1917 (Goostray, 1963), with the first revision a decade later (Committee on Curriculum of the NLNE, 1937).

In the 1930s, the Depression's employment crisis and the generally uncertain times led to a reconceptualization of nursing school curricula as dynamic and progressive rather than static and to emphases on principles of science, the development of teaching, and more democratic (than the traditional autocratic) pedagogies. In essence, students were to be aided in adjusting to nursing and its work (Committee on Curriculum of the NLNE, 1937). As programs became more academic, schools began charging tuition rather than paying students a stipend for ward services. Practical work still dominated the curriculum, but students now attended classes for at least half a year before working regular ward shifts and rotating through different services. Theoretical work was heavily concentrated in the first year (Flood, 1981).

The third and final curriculum guide from the NLNE appeared in 1937 with increased concentration on the community and the inclusion of psychiatry (Kalisch & Kalisch, 1995). The curriculum lasted two and a half to three years, with four weeks vacation each year. About 800 functional learning activities were grouped around the organization and management of the patient's environment to provide physical and mental comfort and well being: personal hygiene of the patient (sick or well); diagnostic and therapeutic measures in which the nurse assisted the physician or carried out procedures directed by him; and community health services involving the care of both individuals and groups. The patient was clearly conceptualized as the focus of nursing efforts (Committee on Curriculum of the NLNE, 1937), although the teaching and settings in which nurses practiced reinforced concentration on the tasks performed, whether those centered on the patient, physician, or institution. According to the Committee on Curriculum of the NLNE (1937), nursing schools were to focus on education and students' educational needs, not the operating needs of the hospitals. The term "pupil" was replaced by "student" to imply active learning and education, rather than training (Flood, 1981). Standards were delineated for allocation of resources, student support and living conditions, teaching, and supervision. Instruction time over the total training period was increased to supplement the approximately 40 hours weekly of "ward practice." Schools were encouraged to share educational resources and opportunities with each other, including their faculty, laboratories, and classrooms (Dolan, 1963).

With its instrumental, if not philosophical, roots firmly planted in the rationalism of scientific medicine, the utilitarianism of hospital labor, and the pull of technological development, it is not surprising that nursing developed a rational technocratic ideology and behaviorist view of student learning. Nursing's earliest pedagogies emphasized problem-solving, formulaic methods, and tools reflecting the neutralized language of technology. Those behavioristic patterns decontextualized and fragmented nursing practice. With behaviorism holding sway, alternative ways of relating to the nursing world were, and still are, typically relegated to the status of tangential abstraction, and thus in large part left unexplored (Hiraki, 1992). The history of nursing and its pedagogies have a strong anti-intellectual cast, with the image of both the nurse and nursing bound up with the idea of technical skill, emotional control, constraint, authority, order and routine, hard work, meticulousness, close supervision and direction, and clearly defined tasks (Aroskar, 1980; Flood, 1981). With a general mandate that nursing and medicine must be kept clearly separate, and the three-year "nurse-administered indoctrination in subordination of nurses to doctors, there was little likelihood that nurses would challenge physicians' prerogatives" (Flood, 1981, p. 15).

Despite the goal of professional standing for the discipline, pressure was strong to keep the basic training school model (which served the goals of hospitals rather than the discipline) *and* to upgrade the discipline to professional educational status. By 1932, an Association of Collegiate Schools of Nursing was established to promote nursing education at the college level, as well as to encourage nursing-relevant research (Hamilton, 1992). Esther Lucille Brown's (1948) book recommending that basic schools of nursing be placed in colleges and universities rather than hospitals illustrated the dialectic. Concurrently, however, the Ginzberg Report, focusing on nursing shortages rather than on education per se, advised prophetically that professional nurses be profiled according to whether they were prepared at the baccalaureate level, were registered nurses who had graduated from 2-year programs, or were practical nurses who had graduated from 1-year programs (Hamilton, 1992; Kelly, 1985). That model, fostered by the proliferation of junior and community colleges in the 1950s, essentially describes the history of nursing education since that time. Three levels of entry (via a baccalaureate degree, an associate degree, or a traditional diploma from a nurse training program) were accommodated by length, type, and depth of program. Today, the Registered Nurse (RN) workforce is composed of at least 27% with diplomas from nurse training programs, 32% with associate degrees, 31% with bachelor degrees in nursing, and 10% with

master's degrees or doctorates (Bednash, 2000). In recent years, enrollment in bachelor's degree nursing programs has been steadily declining
(Hawke, 2001). Part of the decrease continues to be attributed to the
fact that there are multiple entry levels into nursing. As vague as the
differences among entry levels are, the fact that there is typically little or
no pay differential for the baccalaureate-prepared nurse communicates
clearly (Hawke, 2001). Men are a bit better represented in BSN than
AD programs, but still constitute less than a tenth of the total number
of all nurses in the United States.

Only after the Second World War did basic nursing education move
to a significant extent into colleges and universities. The same time period saw the split of registered nurse education into the technical ADN
(the Associate Degree Nurse trained at junior or community colleges)
and the professional BSN (the nurse with a "baccalaureate of science
in nursing" degree with college preparation). The ADN curricula builds
on a high school diploma and the tuition for the two-year programs
is minimal. Course work was limited to the lower division levels. The
graduates are prepared for skilled nursing roles in structured settings,
as well as to take the state licensure examination (NCLEX-RN), and
they meet requirements for an associate degree.

Concentrated in the upper division, BSN curricula gradually has
come to resemble those of other four-year professional majors (Hamilton, 1992). By meeting the college requirements for the academic baccalaureate degree as well as the requirements for taking and passing
the RN licensure exam (the same NCLEX-RN as noted above), BSN
graduates end up prepared to provide skilled, theory-based, and re-
search-fostered nursing care based on any level of need from that of
individuals to populations. In addition to the generic or standard baccalaureate program, a number of programs were developed to build on
the ADN toward achieving a BSN, usually with the working nurse in
mind. There are now also numerous master's degree programs and
tracks to prepare BSN nurses for practice in clinical specialties at advanced levels or for careers in education, administration, or consultation
(Hamilton, 1992). Recent decades have seen the rapid proliferation of
more than fifty doctoral programs in nursing. Some of those (such as
the Ph.D.) focus on academic concerns such as research, while others
are more clinically oriented (e.g., the DSN or ND). Concern is brewing
about levels of academic preparation in this new "orgy of expansion."

It is in large part lip service that idealizes "more" nursing education, since graduates of all RN programs are routinely hired to do the same work. That the nurse with more theoretical background might do the work differently from the technically trained nurse does not typically provide an impetus to differentiate their roles in the managerial eye, since both nurses are licensed to meet the same minimum standards of care. However, tension remains between the two contenders (the associate degree and baccalaureate programs, as few diploma programs exist today) over educational curricula. For many educators and administrators, the fact that students from all levels of entry take the same basic licensing examination justifies the idea of the curricula remaining markedly similar at all current levels of entry and practice and, with the exception of additional focus on patient teaching, amazingly similar to the original curriculum. Once instituted, nursing's pedagogies seem to have been only perfunctorily critiqued and to have undergone little profound modification.

In the late 1960s, a joint American Nurses Association and National League for Nursing national commission probed the intricacies of the supply and demand of nurses, their roles and function, and their careers and educations. That final report called for more government funding for nursing research and for states to take an active role in planning nursing education (National Commission for the Study of Nursing and Nursing Education, 1970). Despite this and other studies, little has changed. In 1965, the ANA adopted the position that the minimum preparation for technical level nursing would be the associate degree and for the professional nurse the baccalaureate, with the resolution that by 1985, the latter would be the minimum preparation for entry into professional nursing practice (American Nurses' Association, 1965). That end was not achieved and there is no evidence that such an initiative will ever be met.

The historical continuity of nursing's pedagogical trajectory is collaborated by critical examination of nursing textbooks over time, which, as cultural commodities, reveal the seldom-explicated ideological and political ideas embedded in the curriculum. Hiraki's (1992) thorough analytical scrutiny of the most often used books disclosed strong, taken-for-granted metaphors that clearly communicate the meaning of nursing practice as mechanistic and wedded to technical rationality. While professional nursing claims to be theory-driven, a positivistic separation of nursing's values from the facts of its primarily technical practice seriously challenges the use of theory in that practice (Hiraki, 1992). The demand for faster production of more RNs, together with the fact that students have many other choices today (which makes it hard for nursing programs to count on getting those who may be best prepared), have further lured nursing education at all levels into technical and practice-oriented schooling.

Nursing's drift into claiming to value one thing but doing another reflects the pedagogical facility with which students can adapt to situations that differ from those intended or that even work against learning. For instance, when there is a heavy investment in testing, science-based, task-oriented behaviors become the basis for understanding care and caring (Diekelmann, 1992). Subtle but unsettling conflicts emerge when nurses, knowing and believing that care should be more than the application of problem-solving methods, experience fact and value as dichotomous in everyday practice. Nursing textbooks often speak to holistic and humanistic aspects of nursing care while failing to present clearly how those broad philosophies or the client's participation might be effectively integrated into nursing process. Over time, nursing has risked further paradigmatic paralysis by limiting itself primarily to theory generated by research predicated only on the physical sciences. Despite ideals of holism and caring, nursing has been prevented from achieving these ideals from its earliest days (when curricular models emphasized training and technique) until the present by the primacy and authority of the empirical-analytical tradition of science (National League for Nursing, 1988).

In sum, in today's rapidly changing and ever more diverse and complex medical and healthcare delivery systems, more than half of all Registered Nurses have no academic degrees above the associate level (David, 2000). A standardized lack of preparation locks nurses into a manual, nontheoretical, lower-class practice that remains, for most, perpetually basic, service-oriented and, at best, quasi-professional. In failing to render the academic preparation of nurses equal to that of other health practitioners, nursing continues to exclude itself from full participation in medical and healthcare discourse.

The Training Mirror

In 1872, the first American nurse training program opened with five probationers at the New England Hospital for Women and Children in

Boston, offering a 12-month graded program in scientific nursing (Hamilton, 1992; Roberts, 1954). Based on an authoritative organizational system, a superintendent directed probationers and student nurses who were learners rather than servants. Physicians lectured on medical and surgical topics (Kalisch & Kalisch, 1995). As in many programs until the 1970s, married and older women were excluded. Schools adopted the Nightingale pledge (which reflected the ideals of the Victorian era) and used textbooks penned by physicians with or without the collaboration of nurses. A minute proportion of learning was devoted to theory and the rest to practice (Kalisch & Kalisch, 1995). The developing American programs differed from Nightingale's programs in England by not being financially endowed, a highly significant fact. Having no independent financial backing, the survival of American nurse training programs was dependent upon schools agreeing to provide nursing service in return for the clinical experience hospitals provided. Overall, nurse training involved maternalistic apprenticeship programs that differed little from the paternalistic systems common to preindustrial times (Ashley, 1976).

The nurse training school was a total institution; social boundaries between private and public life were virtually nonexistent (Goffman, 1961). Young women "entering nursing" were separated from family and community to live under rigid discipline and surveillance by pervasive female authorities (Flood, 1981; Goffman, 1961; Melosh, 1982). Each program determined its own standards of enrollment and practice (Lewenson, 1996). The training routine, initially so rigorous that significant numbers of students fell ill or left, was toned down and lengthened (Kalisch & Kalisch, 1995). A probationary period tested commitment to and fitness for nursing (Flood, 1981). After a successful probation, capping added prestige and responsibilities. Finally, positions based on the idea of caring for the "hospital family" through economic production (services) and loyalty to the institution were created for the students upon graduation. Everyday nursing involved "taking care" of patients (implying measures of physical comfort and assistance with personal hygiene), assisting physicians, and maintaining order and an acceptable rhythm in the ward (Flood, 1981).

All of the departments in the hospital (wards, surgical suites, storerooms, and kitchens) depended on nurses' presence around the clock. It was they who provided care and treatment, did the housekeeping, dispensed drugs, supervised diets and the kitchen, and took care of patients and physicians. In many cases, these "nurses" were really students.

While women apprentices and hospitals could have contractual relationships, there was a legal vacuum around apprenticeship, the practices of which relied not on law but custom. Institutions agreed to provide room, board, and instruction, while applicants agreed to comply with the authority and nonnegotiable rules of the hospital and school (Ashley, 1976). There was full acknowledgment by those who ran them that the main reason for maintaining nursing schools was the monetary value of student nurse services. Meanwhile, political, social, educational, and especially economic factors prevented nurses' organizations from having any major effect on the apprenticeship system of education. In the mid-1930s, nearly 30% of salaried nursing teaching staff had not finished high school (although most of their students had), and few faculty had any college education.

Nurses neither escaped the psychological effects of subordination to the medical profession nor resisted the regimentation of hospital training (Ashley, 1976). Between 1890 and 1920, their training supported the development of nursing as skilled paid labor rather than as a household responsibility (which is what it had been when Nightingale published *Notes on Nursing*). Over time, nursing became increasingly science oriented as new medical knowledge led to treatment of contagious diseases using precise isolation techniques based on the germ theory rather than on the old principles of good housekeeping that had originally shaped nursing activities (Melosh, 1982). Diploma programs graduated more new nurses than associate and baccalaureate programs combined until 1971, despite the professional versus technical debate having begun in 1912 when prominent nurses, criticizing the apprenticeship approach and the wide variability of standards in nursing programs, pressed for a standardized academic curriculum separate from ward service and for uniform requirements for admission (Melosh, 1982). However, in the absence of alternative mechanisms for funding nursing education until nearly the middle of the twentieth century (Ashley, 1976), hospital nurse training programs prevailed.

The Hospital Training Mirror

Hospitals, quickly finding it profitable to proliferate nurse training schools, were free to do so without assessing "the adequacy of their clinical and other resources for teaching nursing" (Roberts, 1954, p. 164). Nursing leaders and the *American Journal of Nursing* deplored "renegade" nurses who supported the unchecked growth of schools by setting up programs that did not conform to the Nightingale ideal (Melosh, 1982). When the 1910 Flexner Report revealed substandard schools of medicine and resulted in closing many of them, nursing leaders proposed a similar study for nursing. The resulting Winslow-Goldmark Report strongly supported education beyond basic preparation for public health nurses, supervisors, and instructors (Goldmark, 1923). However, the push for more education had little impact since hospitals needed the labor that students provided (Flood, 1981; Glass & Brand, 1979). To hospitals, nursing students were a self-perpetuating source of labor. When graduates left to do private duty, hospital superintendents recruited new students to cover the work. Meanwhile, as physicians embraced the tenets of scientific medicine with its increasing reliance on laboratory work, advanced surgery, and clinical diagnosis, many of the traditional roles associated with medical practice fell to nurses (Flood, 1981; Hiestand, 2000; Kalisch & Kalisch, 1995). By 1930, hospitals were hiring more graduate nurses for supervisory positions, although in many places students continued in both staff and supervisory positions (Melosh, 1982).

The nurse training situation was out of control. Nursing was losing ground educationally in comparison to other fields such as social work, physical therapy, home economics, and library work, which women gained more professional status by entering (Garrison, 1979; Grey, 1931; Lobove, 1965). Nursing leaders had for years tried to gain control over nurse training and to garner support for increased academic exposure for student nurses, but the training programs remained securely in the hands of hospital managers and boards of trustees (Ashley, 1976; Melosh, 1982). In the 1930s, apprentices got "direct supervision" only an average of "eleven minutes per ten-hour day," which surely must call into question the quality of care and treatment that was being provided—although those were not the priorities in hospitals (Ashley, 1976, p. 89).

The ambiguous nature of nursing's social position was firmly established early on. An ongoing legal debate involved the status of student nurses as women training for an occupation rather than active laborers, for by 1901 student nurses were listed in the census as employees (Melosh, 1982). The U.S. Census counted both students and graduates as trained nurses (Flood, 1981). The NLNE campaigned for change that would recognize student status without the aid of legislation. The belief prevailed, however, that nurses learned what they needed to know by doing

doing (Ashley, 1976). Over time, it dawned on nursing educators and leaders that they were powerless when it came to improving conditions in hospital schools. Since most of the problems in apprenticeship were embedded in the conflict between labor and management, they could have been more effectively dealt with by the labor movement than by nursing. However, hospital management remained outside the bounds of public authority, controlled its own policies, and generally did not consider the quality of services provided by its labor force a priority. Although none of the facts of hospital organization and authority necessarily prevented nursing from forming a union or otherwise utilizing the labor tactics of the day to help resolve its issues, no serious attempt was made to do that. Until the 1930s, there was virtually no differentiation between services rendered by trained nurses and those of immature and inexperienced students. Likewise, there was little attention paid to staffing patterns or the quality of care provided by women who worked up to fifteen hours a day. 15 hrs/ day

Nurse training schools were tied to hospitals for funding, but since many hospital administrators and training school superintendents were trained nurses, it was often nurses themselves who perpetuated the apprenticeship system in direct challenge to the values of a more professional ideology. Even as health sciences and nursing became more complex, nurses held tenaciously to economic-based and commercial apprenticeship as the only "real" way of learning nursing (Ashley, 1976). To this day, nursing has not abandoned its commitment to practice, allowing theory to become separated from application and praxis and giving way recurrently to traditional technical training and practice models. Like hospital administrators, nurse training program faculty generally saw no reason to pay graduates for services that students would perform in exchange for room, board, training, and a small stipend (Melosh, 1982). Nurses were not taught to question the moral or social implications of the system, or encouraged to develop intellectually through more liberal or general educations. In the early days of nursing's pedagogies, students were homogeneous in age and often in background, and learned a single method of nursing (Flood, 1981). Even during the United States' flood of immigration around the turn of the twentieth century, when education was strictly segregated by sex, the ability to enroll in programs of higher education depended in large part on the capacity to conform to (or at least to espouse) standard American norms and values (Parrillo, 1990). Institutional routines and idiosyncracies were taken for granted as the norm ("Graduates versus students," 1933). When most trained nurses came from middle-class backgrounds there was little need to include instruction in the social graces in the apprenticeship programs. Over time, the class origins of students became more heterogeneous, although liberal education and social skills remained absent from most curricula and communication and interpersonal skills often suffered as a result. It was a costly pattern. Professional comportment was demanded of individuals engaged in other profession-aspiring socialization experiences.

Nursing and hospitals, having established a symbiotic relationship so enmeshed that many observers no longer differentiated the two institutions, faced very real problems during the 1930s when changes on both fronts prompted reconsideration of the bond. Medicine was changing to the extent that nursing students could no longer be depended upon to have experience and knowledge adequate to the situation. More hospitals were hiring experienced graduate nurses and could not maintain training schools without fiscal benefit to themselves (Melosh, 1982). At the same time, nursing organizations were pressuring for reduced use of nursing students as laborers, the presence of instructors for both classroom and clinical skills, and standardization in state board requirements. (By 1923, all states required licensure by examination, but it was not until nearly 1950 that they all used the same test [Hamilton, 1992]). The crux of the problem was that the nurse training schools *were* the hospital nursing departments (Flood, 1981).

The functional system was both ungraded and piecemeal, with nurses doing whatever work needed to be done at a given time. Students did routine work during the majority of all three years of training time (Flood, 1981). The new case or patient assignment method of the 1930s called for a nurse to be responsible for all the work that needed to be done for a set of patients. Despite many pro-case assignment arguments, nursing supervisors had compelling arguments for maintaining the functional approach—for example, that physical tasks were accomplished in less time using a functional approach. Plus, staffing practices did not allow for more than routine work during evenings and nights (Ewing, 1935; Hrebinak, 1974; Jensen, 1942). Nursing's case method, with the nurse seeing the world more from the patient's than the hospital's perspective, included both tasks and intangibles (Flood, 1981). With the threat to routinized order resonating through the wards, the efficiency of the old functional approach kept even ardent proponents of the case method quiet for years (Ham, 1932; Sellow, 1930; Wayland, McManus & Faddis, 1944; Wetzel, 1936).

Most nurse graduates took hospital jobs primarily because there were few other options (Flood, 1981). Many women worked outside the home only until they married, and all working women had limited work opportunities outside their homes—but, among those roles that required training, they met the fewest limits in teaching and nursing. Social change and need pushed nurses into staff nursing jobs as fast as hospitals created them—most often in the same hospital in which the nurses trained. After the late 1930s, most nurses never left the hospitals, but merely transitioned from being students to being employees in them (Melosh, 1982). From the perspective of nursing's pedagogies, reshaping training schools into genuine educational institutions would have required not only new curricula, but sources of student time and teaching resources that seemed impossible to attain (Flood, 1981).

The Counting, Legitimating, and Organizing Mirror

The United States seems to perennially have both a shortage and an excess of nurses. By the late 1920s, it was obvious that the training schools were oversupplying nurses and that efforts to professionalize nursing were not going well. Nursing was urged to cut back on its programs, as medicine had, by halving its number by 1926. Instead, schools kept pumping out nurses. Existing more to provide nursing service than to train nurses, the schools exposed students first to inadequate or nearly nonexistent academic arrangements and then to underemployment. The superabundance of trained nurse graduates could not be absorbed; graduates could not get positions already filled cheaply by students.

Between 1873 and 1893, superintendents of nurse training programs and nursing leaders organized to promote quality education, legal status for training, and improved working conditions (Lewenson, 1996). The developing associations paralleled those of the middle-class and professional groups of the time. After graduating from nurse training programs, women often found themselves isolated while working alone on private duty cases. To retain or regain the close connections of their nurse training days, alumnae groups proliferated (Lewenson, 1996). In addition to alumnae groups, membership in women's clubs, suffrage organizations, temperance leagues, charities, civic reform groups, and collegiate alumnae groups brought together many reform-minded, educated women into potentially powerful coalitions that often functioned as political strongholds (Ehrenreich & English, 1978). Meanwhile, however, the general public constrained nursing's progress by clinging to stereotypes of nursing as domestic service, a rehearsal for motherhood, an occupation that one could enter at any level of preparation and then leave and reenter at will, and a natural function that, since it was thought to be based on intuition and natural inclination, needed little education and should surely avoid "over-education."

In 1903, North Carolina was the first state to institute nurse registration (Kalisch & Kalisch, 1995). However, strong political opposition by medical organizations slowed the enactment of nationwide nurse licensure laws. Since many believed that the goal of state registration of nurses to protect the public from untrained nurses would never be achieved without women being able and willing to vote for it, by 1912 the two oldest national nursing organizations officially decided to support women's suffrage (Lewenson, 1996). Suffrage for women was radical because it attacked the distinction between public and private, with women being limited to the latter realm (Cott & Pleck, 1979). But many women believed naively that once they had the vote, equality with men—in public and in private—would be nearly automatic.

While progress was slow, the score of years between the Spanish-American War and the declaration of war on Germany in 1917 saw relative advancement for nursing with states securing nurse practice acts, the NLNE upgrading nursing education, and public health improving social and health conditions. Four universities developed courses in public health nursing for graduate nurses (Roberts, 1954). By the 1930s, some nurse training programs began to use local colleges for first-year nursing science courses (Flood, 1981). The few collegiate nursing programs attracted upwardly mobile nurses (Oates, 1938; Petry, 1937; "Universities and nursing education," 1934) and allowed nursing faculty to concentrate on teaching nursing (Flood, 1981). Yet nursing's recruitment appeal remained congruent with the dominant cultural ideals of womanhood—through nursing, a woman would be serving humanity and gaining practical preparation for marriage and motherhood (Bastable, 1979). Meanwhile, the nursing associations struggled to institute and govern the accrediting of programs and continued to have no control over the numbers of nurse training schools (Melosh, 1982). Existing accreditation criteria led to the endorsement of less than 20% of hospital training schools (Committee on the Grading of Nursing Schools, 1931; Flood, 1981; Melosh, 1982). Abraham Flexner's Carnegie-funded report of the inadequate conditions in medical schools had led to reform of medical education between 1910 and 1920, by which time medical education was firmly established as a university discipline with definite educational standards. "Flexner-like" studies were done with Carnegie funds in legal, dental, and teacher education, but not in nursing (Kalisch & Kalisch, 1995). It was 1949 before all accrediting activities were unified into a single nursing agency (Dreves, 1963).

Striving for professionalization, nursing leaders asked why training schools were the handmaidens of hospitals, and why nursing education was not tax supported as was education for medicine, law, and engineering. Yet, with the exception of Lavinia Dock, nursing leaders rarely implicated society's deeply embedded male bias as relevant to occupations considered gendered (Glass & Brand, 1979). Dock's understanding of social process extended to seeing how gender and class in European American society were confounded. She complained of the lack of self respect nursing manifested in its willing commercialization and in its failure to achieve professional stature, to become a public conscience, to take positions on societal questions, to inspire the public to fear low standards, or to resist the changes that befell it (Dock, 1903; Glass & Brand, 1979). But Lavinia Dock aside, it seems that nursing has seldom critiqued its own social context. Perhaps this is to be expected, given nurses' lack of opportunity and preparation for the study of social process. Their discipline being generally shaped more by societal and medical trends than by themselves, nurses acted collectively only in response to legislative attempts to control their practice (Glass & Brand, 1979). Unsuccessful efforts to build coalitions of nurses working toward improved and standardized education, accreditation of schools, and definitions of practice led many to conclude that women were powerless without the vote. Yet until nursing leaders finally concluded in 1910 that woman suffrage would directly benefit them, there was no official support of suffrage by nursing organizations (Lewenson, 1996).

The Public Nurse Mirror

As hospitals mushroomed in the early twentieth century, health problems kept pace in the rapidly growing cities teeming with migrants from rural America and other countries. The societal response, swathed as it was in reform, was the Progressive Era. The Sheppard-Towner Act, which was widely supported by women voters, was hailed as the first outcome of female suffrage in 1921 and led to public programs centered on maternal and child health clinics, kindergartens, and protective codes (Kalisch & Kalisch, 1995; Rothman, 1978). Settlement house workers' ideas about children led to a delivery of healthcare that was less medical than social in venue, although the emphasis on domesticity remained intact (Rothman, 1978). The mission of public schools was redefined to develop the entire child in relation to his family and neighborhood. Visiting nursing associations, settlement organizations, and the sanitary movement swept through epidemic-prone urban areas. By 1912, trained nurses visited schools, clinics, factories, and homes; enforced safe water standards; and argued for lighting, garbage removal, and improved tenement housing. Red Cross nurses traveled with the Chautauqua vaudeville entertainers to encourage the hiring of county nurses. District (later public health) nurses taught health promotion and disease prevention measures, working directly in the community rather than out of hospitals (Lewenson, 1996; Melosh, 1982; Rothman, 1978). By 1930, although the discreet nurse avoided open diagnosing, the overall screening process included a definite diagnostic function performed by nurses.

The movement to link health and environmentalism gave women a primary part in community health. Case-finding and health education of whole families expanded as tax funding for public health work spread until, by 1926, one fifth of all trained nurses worked in public health (Melosh, 1982). The movement was pervasive enough to be felt in even the most obscure American locales. Focused on disease prevention and health promotion, and organized apart from and somewhat independent of mainstream curative medicine, the public health movement became nursing's most autonomous domain of practice, and (prior to the advent of master's-prepared clinical nurse specialists and practitioners) that closest to being truly professional. With roots in the settlement movement, the public health movement tried to reconcile prevailing social goals of assimilation with respect for ethnic diversity. Preventive healthcare, which had its origins in charity, became more of a concern of the state and then a matter of ensuring national security and productivity. Eventually, tension between the lived, community-based view of health and its increasing bureaucratization eroded the core of public health nursing (Melosh, 1982).

In 1929 the Sheppard-Towner Act was repealed in large part through efforts of the AMA. During the Great Depression and World War II, public health was prominent in national planning, funding, and relief programs (such as the Social Security Act of 1935), although during the wars medical services focused on the military (Melosh, 1982). In 1930, it was estimated that 9% of the nation's graduate nurses worked in public health (Flood, 1981). But during that decade, rationalization overtook public health. Individualized care and expensive home visiting gave way to generalized community services coordinated by health departments and boards of education (Melosh, 1982). And with public health increasingly medical in tone, nursing became less autonomous. The action reflected private medicine's increasing specialization (Melosh, 1982) and the recurrent expectation that men are professionals and women technicians.

The Conflicted Professionalizing Mirror

From a critical perspective, autonomy refers to the ability to come to terms with constraints imposed on oneself by having internalized self-limiting ideas (Allen, 1987). Professional autonomy that seeks to routinize the quality of care conflicts with bureaucratic control seeking to routinize efficiency (Kleinman, 1995). Historically, it seems autonomy cannot be tolerated in more than one area. Traditional notions of women as being inferior to men were internalized along with the social hubris of twentieth-century progressivism, the age of educated motherhood, and then new images of women as "wife-companions" (Rothman, 1978). As birth control became an explicit issue, Margaret Sanger, a nurse, campaigned valiantly against tremendous opposition for women's right to the knowledge to control their reproduction (Hamilton, 1992; Lerner, 1977). The cosmetic industry boomed; by 1931 women's magazines carried more advertisements for beauty aids than for they did for food.

In the mix of new ideas and old attitudes, nursing was not in a position to monopolize or to make itself indispensable. Furthermore, the nurse seemed always ready to return "where she belonged" when jobs ran low (Ehrenreich & English, 1978). Mainstream America embraced the position that any educated physician was automatically the superior of the apprentice-trained servant/helper nurse (Ashley, 1976). This was so taken for granted that nursing neither seriously examined the repressive reality nor tried to solve the problems that nurses shared with other women (Ashley, 1976). Paying limited attention to the deeper educational and labor issues, few nursing leaders actively promoted nursing participation in the public forum (Dock, 1903). In the United States, nursing's early leadership was shaped by European American women devoted to giving the discipline status in the eyes of the public, medical doctors, and hospital administrators.

For nursing to become respectable work for middle-class women required more than the shedding of pre–Civil War and pre-Nightingale images of low status and low pay for menial, physical, and domestic work done by untrained individuals. Apprenticeship has long been recognized as a mechanism for keeping individuals subject to the will of others (Mill, 1869; Rossi, 1970; Tulloch 1989) and apprenticeship in nursing is no exception. Nursing remained a nonthreatening adjunct to the practice of medicine, incongruously settling into a pattern of trying to meet expectations for professional, autonomous behavior and playing traditional feminine, passive roles (Bush & Kjervik, 1979; Lewenson, 1996), even as it was often heard on the side that "nurses did not need an education because the physician had one" (Ashley, 1976, p. 76). The 1920s and 30s saw a proliferation of AMA-appointed committees on nursing. Physicians complained that nurses had too little scientific theory and practical experience to be useful (Flood, 1981). Although they could not agree on what was best for nurses other than that they needed more practical instruction, few physicians doubted that it was their place to decide (Keller, 1932). They simply overrode nurses' professional organizations with their opinion that nursing was a commodity to be used to the advantage of the medical profession and hospitals (Ashley, 1976).

To make matters worse, graduate nurses competed for work with both student nurses and partially trained or untrained women who were encouraged to fill the ranks for very low pay. "Short courses" were offered by various organizations to provide physicians and the public with "nurses" who had less preparation than hospital-trained graduates. Many of these substitutes were dropouts from nursing schools, where the attrition rates were high (Flood, 1981). The notion of subsidiary workers trained for absolute adherence to physicians' orders and cleanliness gained favor among medical and hospital administrators, later producing attendants, aides, assistants, and practical nurses instructed by anyone who cared to create a short course (Ashley, 1976; Flood, 1981). With no practical way of distinguishing among levels of preparation of nurses, consumers usually ended up paying the same rate for any "nurse" label. Nursing was diluted by indistinguishable varieties of "nurses," and the discipline was again devalued as little more than menial women's work. While other groups aspiring to professional status made rapid progress in acquiring a liberal education, nursing was coping with "eight-week courses training housekeepers for the sick, and correspondence courses. No other group claiming to be a profession since 1873 had to contend with such circumstances" (Ashley, 1976, p. 69).

While better than the subsidiary programs, hospital nurse training programs fostered a limiting orientation that emphasized the needs of others; unquestioning loyalty to hospitals; respect for authority; cooperation, obedience, and docility; and a tolerance for poor work conditions and stringent discipline (Ashley, 1976). Independence, innovative problem-solving, and social competencies were asides. Heads of training schools, products of the same narrow pedagogical format, perpetuated the rules and subservience that they had internalized as students. Not surprisingly, nurses' occupational culture valued manual skills, direct involvement with the sick, respect for experience and mistrust of theory, and a replication of the medical hierarchy within the nursing realm. Of all the occupations, nursing is probably the one that has been the most affected by social conceptions of the nature of women as less assertive, creative, and independent than men (Ashley, 1976).

Arguments over nursing's status go back as far as the first rejection of the sentimental and uncompensated "angel of mercy" image in favor of nursing as a realization of self with a professional identity. Depicted as a vocational calling or "merely a gainful occupation" (Melosh, 1982, p. 23), nursing has also been represented as a discipline cursed by a context that imposed intractable cultural contradictions. It has been idealized as the epitome of women's *real* work, a sentiment made complete by the suggestion that nurses hide behind a facade of professional demeanor merely to enhance the ability to "take things as they come" (Melosh, 1982, p. 56). Blocked from professional status by being all of those things, nursing's only constant has been being more reactive than proactive on behalf of the discipline. When hospitals recognized that nurse training programs were costing them money, apprenticeship became obsolete. At the same time, it was acknowledged that nurses needed more theoretical training to practice in changing contexts where patient care had become more complex with expanding therapeutics (Melosh, 1982). The stage was set for more academic nursing education.

What prevented the needed transformation from occurring when nursing education was no longer relegated to apprenticeship training and valued only as labor? The extent to which lack of male support affected nursing's progress in terms of increased power, prestige, and wealth is questionable (Glass & Brand, 1979). Clearly, the advance of selected professions was supported by male-dominated institutions. However, nursing clearly helped maintain its own subordination. For example, by the mid–twentieth century, nursing was setting standards of practice and nationally accrediting its schools of nursing even as educators argued vigorously about time spent learning the "theory of nursing" detracting from the quality of actual patient care. The discipline burdened itself with multiple, often competing, professional organizations. Although some nurses have done much to extricate themselves from semi-professional status and stereotyped "women's work," many others have consistently succumbed to institutionalized social expectations that preclude leaving either behind. In sum, nursing failed to take command of those matters within their jurisdiction that might have worked toward rather than against its professionalization: numbers of school and students, standards of education and practice, levels of entry into practice, and sources of competition. When nursing finally did make efforts to set limits, the boundaries were typically unenforceable due to the actions of others both outside the discipline and within.

At the inception of organized nursing, nurses were in many ways the equals of physicians in their training and contributions to the healthcare of society. However, over time, as the medical establishment coalesced and strengthened, the gendered groups became more politically and economically disparate. Nurses did not have a capacity for influencing society or being recognized by it, and relatively little was done to alter either circumstance. While that traditional lack of equality had an impact on the development of the discipline, newer contradictions precluded full professionalism. For instance, wanting nursing staff to be available at all hours and to work as long as a situation demands implies professional obligations, not those of hourly laborers. Yet the same nursing service is expected to exude unquestioning subservience as physicians give orders and nurses carry them out. Overall, nursing tried to change its historical trajectory toward a more professional direction *while* maintaining its "artifice of ladylike powerlessness" (Ashley, 1976, p. vi). It is not surprising that efforts to have it both ways have failed.

The eventual division of nursing practice and education into a hierarchy based on theoretical expertise (that is, into professional and technical categories) further removed nurses from potential for gaining broader support through strategies such as trade unionism or more inclusive educational programs (Melosh, 1982). Over time, smaller proportions of nurses came with the educational advantages of the middle or upper middle classes. With limited backgrounds in liberal education, which the commercial interests of hospitals controlling nursing education did nothing to redress, nurses often lacked the social and political skills needed to support potential professional status and prestige. Nurses have been soundly criticized for lack of knowledge, lack of manners, and deficiencies in professional preparation, as well as for being unable to provide effective community service or improvement in patient care. There was, in sum, virtually no way to get beyond "semi-profession" status. Even highly educated nurses were discriminated against in the continuing subordination to physicians—a situation exacerbated by higher education for nurses being at times eschewed by many nurses themselves. Overall, the story of the largest group in the healthcare and medical industries has remained, in large part, one in which its protagonists have been rendered anonymous and relegated to secondary status, and in which the image of nursing has been neither particularly positive nor assertive, but shaped by its role in the workplace and reinforced by its pedagogical traditions.

The Working and Military Mirrors

The human condition of labor is life itself.
Arendt, 1958, p. 7

Women's occupations (such as nursing, school teaching, childcare, the manufacture of textiles and clothing, domestic service, and prostitution) have typically been viewed as extensions of household responsibilities and presumed to fit women's physical, psychological, and intellectual capacities. However, reflecting American society over time, women's work also diversified. Change came slowly in the schooling of nurses with fluctuating notions about the value of submissiveness and nurturance, while the service expected of nurses expanded rapidly. In 1922 the first report to include studies of institutional nursing revealed the common practice of permitting far more orders to be written for nursing procedures than could be effectively executed by available nursing staffs (Roberts, 1954). The routine failure of administrators of nursing services and hospitals to do anything about resolving the deficit has profoundly affected decades of nursing care and nurses' morale (Roberts, 1954). The only response to impossible workloads has been ongoing toleration by nurses, nursing administrators, and nursing faculty. As new roles evolved in healthcare, tasks were not so much dispersed among other positions as added to the nursing repertoire (Kalisch & Kalisch, 1995).

The nineteenth-century ethos of domestic nursing was preserved by freelance, private-duty nursing. When the growing middle class found urban life prevented them from relying on extended family to do nursing chores, they often hired private-duty nurses for home care. Paid by families, such nurses were on duty virtually around the clock (Lewenson, 1996; Roberts, 1954). As hospitals gained popularity and fewer infectious diseases wreaked epidemic fluctuations of risks and needs, shorter units of nursing time were needed. Nursing's tumultuous struggle with hospitals for staff-nurse employment was essentially won by organized nursing by the late 1930s, but nurses did not flock to the floor-nursing positions as they did to administrative or public-health work (Flood, 1981). Although hospital nursing provided variety and an opportunity to keep up with changes, the volume of work and the quality of supervision resulted in high turnover. The ANA viewed the unions as competitors for nurse affiliation and resented their involvement in nursing's efforts to "educate" hospitals into changing (Flood, 1981, p. 292; "Meetings of the Board of Directors," 1938; "Union membership? No!," 1938). Either it was not suggested at that time that some of the more routine nursing tasks be relegated to another category of worker or the possibility was screened out of the published literature. In any event, it does not appear that general staff nurses were eager to rid themselves of those menial tasks that are now tangential to nursing care (Flood, 1981; Sellow, 1930).

Although Nightingale had made it clear that nurses must be paid fairly for their labors (Bishop & Goldie, 1962), wages were low and prestige limited because the employers of nurses were not willing or able to compete in labor markets for the services of men (Brownlee &

Brownlee, 1976). Graduate nurses increasingly sought hospital staff-nurse jobs, but demand (and compensation) remained slack. Those nurses who worked outside the hospital were chronically underemployed (Ashley, 1976). During the Great Depression, paid work was scarce and most women lost ground, many returning to the home while men filled the limited numbers of jobs available.

Meanwhile, with the Depression's general economic collapse, poor people simply did without medical assistance (Kalisch & Kalisch, 1995). Aides and practical nurses weathered the economic times better than graduate nurses did, since hospitals tended to employ graduates at the same salaries paid to subsidiary personnel.

The proliferation of training schools imposed continuous overcrowding and competition in the occupation, which the Depression only made more obvious. In sum, the Depression functioned primarily as a convenient excuse to maintain the status quo in nursing education (Glass & Brand, 1979). Nursing's employment problems did not significantly lessen until World War II, when they disappeared—at least temporarily and in terms of job availability (Melosh, 1982).

The end of the Depression brought no reforms of significance for working nurses. Medical sexism and increasing medicocentrism preserved the status quo (Coburn & Willis, 2000; Kleinman, 1995). Job insecurity and a high risk of unemployment were routine, as were high rates of dissatisfaction with pay, work conditions, and prospects of promotion (Ashley, 1976). Most nurses worked to supplement husbands' incomes or, during the war, for patriotic reasons. Overall, however, the period between 1933 and 1952 was probably nursing's most exciting, due to the changes that occurred. A major factor was the Social Security Act. It had an effect on ideas about health and provided an impetus for federal social legislation, including laws that authorized training nurses as public-health workers (Dreves, 1963). Historically, nursing has always had productive links to the military, which proved a major consumer of nursing services. World War I was an endurance test for schools of nursing. Leaders resisted government attempts to shorten training courses and remained involved as women (who did not yet have the vote) sustained the economy and did the work normally reserved for men, including physicians (Glass & Brand, 1979). The war left unresolved the highly controversial issue of preparing and employing nurses' aides while many nurses were overseas and nursing staffs were depleted. By 1920, after the war and the influenza epidemic, the United States faced a shortage of about 55,000 active nurses (Kalisch & Kalisch, 1995).

World War II resolved the nurses' aides issue (that is, whether to substitute aides for nurses) but left the question of conscripting nurses dangling because nurses rose to the occasion and managed to meet the demands of both military and civilian needs without it. Of the nation's nurses eligible for military service, more than 40% volunteered for military service (Roberts, 1954). When World War II began, "there were not enough nurses for peacetime let alone war service" (Dreves, 1963, p. 20). Subsequent defense spending supplied supplementary courses and crash programs for nursing, the most notable being the Cadet Nurse Corps, initiated in 1943. This both produced large numbers of trained nurses and increased the public's awareness of the need for federally supported education for nurses (Glass & Brand, 1979; Kalisch & Kalisch, 1995). By 1944, most students in accredited schools came under the U.S. Cadet Nurse Corps, through which the U.S. Public Health Service subsidized 30-month courses. Participating students promised to engage in essential military or civilian nursing for the duration of the war (Kalisch & Kalisch, 1995; Melosh, 1982; Roberts, 1954). In 1942, a new act provided for relative rank for all members of both the Army and Navy Nurse Corps, giving them the same pay and allowances as officers of comparable rank without dependents in other branches of the services. This served as an important recruitment factor, although permanent, commissioned rank was not provided for until 1947 (Roberts, 1954). By 1948, 124,000 nurse cadets had been graduated and the nursing resources of the institutions that had participated in the program were greatly increased (Roberts, 1954). Over the five-year program, each cadet cost the government a scant $1360 for training (Roberts, 1954). The Cadet Nurse Corps clearly dramatized the military's recognition of nursing as an essential service and verified the advantages of funding nursing education. Nursing leaders worked on attracting more federal monies after the war, particularly for baccalaureate education, while the AMA unfailingly lobbied against such action (Melosh, 1982).

In 1946, when almost 45,000 nurses were released from military service (Roberts, 1954), only one Army nurse in six returned to her pre-war, civilian nursing position (Kalisch & Kalisch, 1995). The post-war ideology later called "the feminine mystique" urged women to go back to the home rather than to work (Elder, 1958; Kalisch & Kalisch, 1995;

Melosh, 1982), while the poor wages and unsatisfying working conditions of civilian hospitals led nurses to prefer self-sacrifice at home over employment (Ashley, 1976). In 1947, the Hill-Burton Act supported new hospital construction with fully rationalized workforces and increasingly stratified hierarchy based on wartime nursing models (albeit without military rank) (Melosh, 1982). Over time, prepayment health plans, increasing life expectancies, high-speed transportation, medical and pharmaceutical advances, proliferating nursing homes, and changing nursing care all made it easier to gain access to nursing care and to be employed as a nurse (Dreves, 1963). After graduation of the last large class of cadet nurses in 1947, enrollment in accredited nursing schools plummeted—yet programs for nurse's aides and practical nurses proliferated. Never again were as many nurses involved in direct (that is, personal care of individuals, as contrasted with administrative, educational, or other "indirect" roles) nursing care practices performed by registered nurses as before World War II. By 1952, practical nurses and nurses' aides provided most nursing services (Kalisch & Kalisch, 1995).

The Gender, Class and Culture Mirror

It is a fallacy that "The only history is white."
Césaire, 1972, p. 54

The trend may appear linear, with women gaining equality in industrial societies, but it is actually curvilinear because women are *regaining* some of the equality lost in the transition from simple foraging societies to those that are industrialized nation states (Whyte, 1978). Generally, despite wide cultural variations in sex roles and stereotypes, in stratified (that is, nation-state) societies, the aggregate duties, prohibitions, and traits of women relegate them to a lower status than that typical of males. Women have political power and prestige, but it is concentrated in minor offices and womanhood translates into unequal economic relations. As occurs with other oppressed groups (Freire, 1971; Roberts, 2000), women's group consciousness can be viewed as a subculture divided against itself by its informing and restricting ties to the dominant culture. This interdependence between historical continuity and change reveals strengths as well as weaknesses, and enduring values as well as accommodation (Cott, 1972). The legacy of nineteenth-century womanhood was not erased from American culture by the ideological change that shifted allegiances from women's clubs to settlement houses and then personal-interest groups. The familiar domestic tenets were renewed with vigor after World War II, when the 1950s revived the norms of the 1920s and provided the setting for the emergence of the women's liberation movement.

The elemental task of understanding woman's history is replicated in that of nursing, which has always been shaped by phenomena that do not show up much in either nursing or historical records, such as gender differences, class differences, culture and, for many, "race." The same divisions that characterized American society were reflected in schools of nursing. Initially immigrants, Jews, and persons of color were not accepted in nurse training programs, except where the rare quota might endure a token individual from such categories. However, in the twentieth century, American society switched commitments—from a widely shared, largely implicit policy of cultural assimilation (based on the conviction that difference constituted liabilities that should be minimized) to one of more pluralistic tolerance for diversity. With this change, scholarly accounts of histories of nurses of color began to appear (e.g., Carnegie, 1986; Hine, 1989). Whereas previous records of nursing history left out the voices of those nurses not of European descent, born in the United States, and otherwise typical, revised nursing histories are now becoming more inclusive.

Since nursing schools, like hospitals and other medical establishments, were typically racially segregated until well into the 1950s, women of color have always been underrepresented in nursing (Melosh, 1982). Most white suffragists shared society's rarely challenged and strongly predominant racist views in the early twentieth century. A few far-seeing African Americans supported women's suffrage because they understood that sooner or later African Americans would benefit from the fact that Black as well as white women would be entitled to vote (Flexner, 1975). Until the 1960s (and in some cases later), persons of color were often relegated to separate and inferior schools, subjected to various forms of discrimination, and left to their own devices whenever they sought to overcome the racial prejudice affecting both the education of nurses and the provision of healthcare services to members of minority groups. Nonetheless, nursing can boast that it integrated its racially segregated professional organizations before medicine did. Since nurses belong to the American Nurses Association through their state nurses associations, full integration of the organization followed that of the state level groups. As soon as membership in the National Nurses Association was available, the National Association of Colored Graduate Nurses dissolved (Roberts, 1954). On the other hand, nursing education has been criticized for its color-blind perspectives (Barbee, 1993; Hoff, 1994; Jackson, 1993, 1994; Kavanagh, 1988, 1991, 1995; Kavanagh & Kennedy, 1992; Kavanagh, Kennedy, Kohler & Rasin, 1993). In the name of justice but propelled by the expediency of ratio- nality and efficiency, nurses often resort to assuming that social differ- ences (such as race, gender, ethnicity, and economic status) are irrele- vant to and can be ignored in healthcare. Unfortunately, that practice denies experiences that people find meaningful in their lives and advo- cates that everyone be treated in the same way. Effacing difference in the name of efficiency deprives nursing of opportunities to work for social transformation that would be likely to benefit the discipline as well as members of other social categories.

The Confluence of Ideological Mirrors:
Reflections of and on Nursing's Pedagogies

Humans do not ponder or think or know their ownmost determination.
Heidegger, 1999

Any authentic response to "How is it nursing is the way it is?" in- volves interpretations reflecting myriad possibilities and the idea that there are multiple and complex pedagogies (Hernández, 1997). As mir- rors forming a matrix of enveloping space in which culture and history reveal themselves, multiple ideological influences have been recounted in light of their shaping nursing's pedagogies. There are likely many additional ways of looking at patterns of history and culture in the com- pilation of nursing's pedagogies. The reflections coalesce in dialectics ranging from that juxtaposing the good of society with the good of nurs- ing, to others more specific to the history and culture of nursing educa- tion. At every turn there are tensions around decisions presumed to have been made freely, but that reflect hegemonic constraints that often go unrecognized or are accepted as part of some natural process. The fact that nurses often disagree about the issues that shape their disci- pline and work manifests the fragmentation that maintains the status quo. It has been predicted that nursing cannot survive the way it is today

(David, 2000; Hall, 1999; Valiga, 1988). At the very least, the question arises whether the discipline will succumb to its present or transform itself to make a different future.

In nursing, power is seldom exercised in overt and observable ways (Peters, Marshall, & Fitzsimons, 2000), and issues of power and hegemony are rarely confronted. Political and economic realities continually reassert themselves in everyday social relations and activities (Apple, 1988), but nursing has yet to acknowledge its need to overcome patterns established in the past. Perhaps its avoidance pattern is based on common knowledge and research findings of a highly consistent cultural conviction that nurses' work is dirty work, especially when it involves direct contact with the body or body products (Lawler, 1993). To many, nursing skills remain a refinement of the "natural" (biologically determined) aptitudes of women (Gamarnikow, 1978; Lawler, 1993). Because nurses's work hovers so close to traditional women's roles, it is in constant peril of being ignored (Lewin, 1977; Oakley, 1974, 1984). Given the general historical exclusion of women and nurses as significant "knowers" or agents of knowledge, it rings true that understanding nursing requires critically examining "the sources of social power" (Harding, 1987, p. 9).

Nursing's is a particular story in the realm of shared histories of the professions and the other health-related disciplines. Superficially, it is tempting to conclude that nursing is unable to resolve its problems because it has picked and fought its battles naively or inexpertly; was not prepared to defend itself successfully against aggressive professional competition determined to maintain nursing's subservience; failed to recognize or act on opportunities for productive response; or too often declined to confront social issues relevant to the discipline that could have rallied public attention and support. However, it would be more plausible to assume that until nurses change their own consciousness and seize the power of self-definition they cannot expect change from others (David, 2000). The realization of the need for empowerment based on self-efficacy is contingent upon understanding the process of marginalization that, in the dialectic of gender, has ordained the primacy of difference and kept the borders of authority and power intact, rendering nursing the "unequal other."

Marginalized peoples are negatively "different," objectified, closely watched, and not viewed as credible, while marginalization (the peripheralization of a group or individuals by a dominant, central source of power [Hall, 1999]), as a dialectic in itself, exposes both vulnerabilities and strengths in any minority (that is, relatively less powerful) group. Marginalization involves characteristics that distinguish nursing from medicine (Hall, 1999). In nursing, there are blurred boundaries around both status and role; a recognition of a cultural uniqueness that can lead to scapegoating and peripheralization as the "other"; authority that involves access to some but not the most important sources of status, power and wealth; limited collective awareness and organization; and problems that arise from enforced conformity (Hall, 1999). Nursing's resistance to authentic evaluation of its situation has been costly. In nursing, as in other occupations and professions, the goal of reflec-tiveness is the honing of survival skills. However, in nursing, the benefits of such reflection are counterbalanced by the exhaustion that continuous vigilance in a sociopolitically volatile world produces. A collectively muted voice allows expression of experience that is different from the dominant myths about the group, but such expression is accompanied by the risk of being silenced. And there is a liminality that sets nursing apart but also risks further alienating it, given that it is outside the core of the dominant system and its protections and resources (Hall, 1999).

When threatened, nursing tends to circle its wagons in self-protection, to retrench by resorting to technical rationality and behavior-alism rather than embracing its core care-oriented values, and to turn inward. Individuals often accept rather than challenge the limitations of their situations. They also strike out against others who are, as often as not, their nurse peers. Such falling back on traditional practice com-promises reflective discourse as well as constructive change. Frank (2000) provides an exemplar of a nurse's destructive limitations in her story of Diane DeVries, a woman who was born without arms and legs. After years of preparing herself against all odds for a professional role, Ms. DeVries earns a master's degree and a social service job as a dis-charge planner. She performs her job well, but soon is fired from her position because the director of nursing interprets Diane's turning the pages of charts with her lips as a violation of principles of infection con-trol. The fact that ensuing litigation was won by pointing out that turning chart pages with lips posed no greater risk than the common practice of nurses licking their fingers before turning the same pages does little to absolve nursing of its limitations. The point is that, having fallen prey to the passive aggressive pettiness commonly associated with oppressed groups, some nurses allow their or others' practice to be tyrannical, while few see the larger dynamics of which they, their behavior, and their work are a part.

Bound by the insidious pedagogical roots of many historical influences, potent cultural values, and seductive social norms, nursing often experiences new possibilities as unsettling. The discipline's social inertia has long limited its contributions along with the risks of being vulnerable to the manipulations of other occupational groups. In nursing's dearth of meaningful discourse with other disciplines, activities such as putting the notion of human "race" in its place as a social rather than a biological construct (Cohen, 1998; Marks, 1994), authentically advocating for patients' self-determination when technologies of domination limit autonomy (Peters, Marshall & Fitzsimons, 2000), helping society make sense of new (e.g., genetic) hegemonies (Finkler, 2000), or grappling with questions pertaining to women's rights or a more humane society (Benhabib & Cornell, 1987), are typically not considered because they are routinely defined as outside nursing's traditionally practice-oriented purview. The health professions grew out of societal need; their futures depend on their ability to negotiate between the best interests of the consumer and the demands of changing times (Joel, 1988). With nursing more often associated with rigidity than with flexibility or understanding, the future reverberates with unmitigated challenge (Rieger, 2000; White, 2000).

Responding to circumstances and precedent, nursing's pedagogies have leaned more toward training for practice than toward learning through experience or valuing learning in its own right. Nursing's pedagogical blind spots and susceptibility to ideological drift have at times been more realistically critiqued from outside the United States than from within (Lundh, Soder, & Waeness, 1988), which attests both to the difficulty of intra-cultural critique and to the reluctance of nursing to associate nursing's pedagogies with its problems. There are exceptions to the general nonexistence of critiques of U.S. nursing pedagogies generated from within the U.S. such as Jean Watson's (1988), which compares the dire state of nursing curriculum to a irreparably shattered Humpty Dumpty. It is small wonder that endless curricular tweaking has not wrought the needed transformation. Diekelmann (1988) advocates a curricular *revolution*—which she envisions as a long process of transformation ultimately resulting in innovative pedagogical change.

As things stand, nurses both blandly resist and blankly accept the hegemonic forces that shape their practice, and they actively participate—their pedagogies being a primary medium—in perpetuating their second class and marginalized status (David, 2000). Nursing curricula undergo surface-level transpositions but, just as earlier women's roles did not meaningfully change despite major societal commutations, at deeper levels, teaching, learning, and schooling in nursing have sustained markedly little modification. Nursing hesitates to institutionalize real educational differences among its levels of entry, and minimizes the significance of distinctions. Associate degree nurses insist that they are professionals and nurses (including faculty) prepared at professional and graduate levels often generously tolerate the misrepresentation—which does more to lower the status of the latter than it does to enhance that of the former. How is it that few nurses recognize the differences as significant enough to expect them to influence practice?

Nonetheless, it is not by will alone that things happen, for what happens and what *matters* is not entirely up to those who care (Heidegger, 1999). Nursing cannot come to grips with its pedagogical problems or construct its own context for practice until it deals with the societal gender and class politics that profoundly affected it in its beginnings and that continue to influence it today. Managing those will require both recognizing how the discipline systematically deludes itself by ignoring the impact of gender and class in its quest for occupational efficacy, *and* understanding how that subterfuge perpetuates the discipline's quasi-professional mediocrity, limits its freedom and growth, and preserves its marginal status (David, 2000). In nursing, status issues rooted in class and gender function as a neglectful absentee landlord whose disregard allows an insidious drift toward dereliction. Sooner or later, to avoid total obsolescence, nursing will need to give up its dependence on a dysfunctional tradition and broaden its views and possibilities. Meanwhile, culturally and historically, the situation reflects nursing's accommodation of suffusive ideologies not its own. It is not that nursing's mirror is irreparably broken; it is in the reinterpretation of the image reflected that essential new insight and promise of survival dwell. The real question is whether nursing can overcome its subordinate status when its continuing under-education prevents it from recognizing links between it and other levels of education, class, gender, and social position (David, 2000).

The Natural Caring Versus Rational Commodity Paradox

The habit of hearing only what we already understand.
Heidegger, 1971, p. 54

Much of the debate about what nursing is reflects disagreement about whether nature (intuition) or nurture (education) should dominate its pedagogies. Historically, the Western tradition's most significant beliefs about women pertain to their nature, despite it also being argued at times that what is natural is opposed to what is human (Richards, 1980). In nursing, one manifestation of the nature versus nurture controversy is the widely accepted view of nursing practice as both science and art (Spicker & Gadow, 1980). Three common models of nurses include the nurse in the natural role as surrogate mother, the nurse as (trained) technician, and the nurse as (both natural and educated) clinician. In relating to clients, the clinician model challenges the nurse—often without support—to do more than merely replicate the client-physician relationship by playing both a natural role and a clinical role. While nurses are obligated to assist physicians (although the obligation is not reciprocal), they are also required to provide the care necessary to meet the patient's needs. It is that aspect of nursing that distinguishes caring from basic social justice, which by itself can be cold and ruthless (Katz, Noddings, & Strike, 1999).

Relationships change continuously among health professionals, between providers and consumers, and in society at large (Spicker & Gadow, 1980). Approaches in preparation and practice roles adjust in kind. Although many nursing roles have undergone change more than nursing's pedagogies have, the concept "care" has been retained as integral to clinical nursing practice (Greenleaf, 1988). The intangibility of caring in a materialistic world creates endless pedagogical challenge. In nursing education, even when students ceased being exploited in apprenticeships, it remained unclear whether the pedagogical ideal involved their being consumers who contracted to earn credentials, or participants in a learning process in open and caring communities of educators and learners (Carlson & Apple, 1998; De Tornyay, 1991). Historically, most nurse educators were socialized in rigidly disciplined, clearly hierarchical, and minimally intellectual hospital training programs. Today, a different set of pressures—the exigencies of cost containment—has encouraged the use of factory-like models of educating in colleges and universities. Industrialized culture conspires against open and humanistic approaches in pedagogy as much as it supports the technicity that shapes much of nursing's work.

Generally, nursing has not opened itself to mindfully engaged dialogue about caring and its worth. The stated goals of nursing and those manifested in the institutions in which nursing is routinely practiced greatly differ. In fact, in the care versus commodity discussion, both nurses and nursing resist being claimed by the core of the discipline's meaning—if that core is caring, as it is often claimed to be the case. There are multiple realities and ideals, but no consensus about what nursing really is and does. Over time, the discipline has allowed itself to be subsumed by the dominant discourse of rationality. Yet, in its dialectical system of values is found the source of its distress: nursing lacks the strength of affiliation (in Heideggerian terms, the joining) to create and sustain a wholeness of its disparate values of caring and technical rationality.

This ambiguity and ambivalence, in combination with nursing's status issues, unwieldy numbers, and diversity of levels of entry and roles, has taken a heavy toll on the discipline's management of its limited autonomy and professionalization. Nursing has not dealt effectively with institutionalized, strongly genderized "glass ceilings" that compromise access to societal resources (that is, prestige, power, and wealth), and lead to devaluation by many of caring as a goal. Explanations for the perennial shortages of nurses (despite the proliferation of schools) usually fall back on the "nature" of women. Common convictions persist about it being "natural" that women be domestic, hold jobs rather than build careers, work outside the home only sporadically, and use nursing as a basis for procuring a husband and caring for a family. However, historically, nursing shortages have as much resulted from as been alleviated by the mass production of credentialed graduates, while pragmatic working problems have not been resolved and the conflicting values of the discipline persist.

Far too little emphasis has been placed on the incentives nurses have to stay in the field and on the way disincentives (such as horizontal violence [that is, the common infighting expressed through intragroup aggression and competition by oppressed groups (Freire, 1982; Hedin, 1986; Roberts, 1983)], glass ceilings, hierarchical pressures, and status differentials) negatively affect nurses' decision making. In their second class status, nurses are bound to and by the authority and power of the higher class and by the gender hierarchy of a gender-class conscious society (David, 2000). For many, race and ethnicity further confound the situation. But the condition of the nursing labor force has typically been analyzed from the perspective of the medical, hospital, and healthcare industries (usually in an attempt to answer the question of why there are unfilled positions) rather than from the perspective of nurses and their experiences with employment. Some rationalize that more nurses are needed because patients are now sicker, but that does not address the fact that far more attention has been concentrated on the need for nurses in active practice than on the real reasons so few stay there.

Proposals to subsidize nursing education with scholarships and to provide financial incentives to nursing students who agree to work in understaffed locations address symptoms rather than underlying status-ridden problems. Why do many nurses leave nursing practice? Why— no matter what the unemployment rate and no matter how fast nurses are produced—do more than 100,000 nursing jobs remain unfilled (Hosler, 2001)? Why are many people willing to do nearly anything except nursing? And why is it that nurses in the military—where rank is commensurate with ability and time in service, not merely determined by whether one has passed the licensure exam or not—seem more satisfied than nurses in the civilian sphere? Since nurses are more often construed as objects than as participants in healthcare discourse, nursing shortages are typically perceived as inalienable artifacts of numbers. One questions whether a professional organization that considers financial aid to students a long-term solution to the "nursing shortage" (Hosler, 2001)—while leaving history and social process unaddressed— can provide the leadership needed to guide nurses into a self-defined future. Nursing's existence is challenged as never before. The old pedagogical paradigm is paralyzing. Does nursing have the resilience needed, in addition to the understanding and verve, for sociopolitical transformation?

For all of its talk about caring, the most pervasive theme in nursing's pedagogies has been rationality, which permeates nearly every aspect of nursing, beginning with the "nursing process"—the discipline's omnipresent format for linear, quasi-scientific problem-solving. While claiming to be holistic and humanistic, properties that are nourished by inductive ways of thinking, nursing typically teaches and rewards deductive, rationalistic, and positivistic thinking. Habermas's (1979) descriptions of instrumental rationality apply to the development of the understanding of nursing process as a (or *the*) legitimate form of reasoning and the basis for practice. Whether assumption or conviction, this notion reflects the tacit presumption that the adoption of scientific methodology will lead to the transformative professionalization of nursing. It has not. Technology, often understood only in terms of its social value, is more than the application of scientific knowledge, for the ends to which technology are put are inevitably value-laden. Most pronounced among those are the values that predominate in American society: personal autonomy, individuality, materialism and consumerism, efficiency and rationality, active (even aggressive) intervention, a sense of time urgency, and mastery over nature (in lieu of harmony with or acceptance of natural phenomena) (Althen, 1988; Stewart & Bennett, 1991). The strength of those values is reflected in the United States' tolerance of medical and health systems in which treatment and care remain a privilege rather than a right.

America's dominant values and those of its health-related industries tend to devalue the humanistic and holistic aspects of caring (Dossey, Keegan & Guzzetta, 2000; Paterson & Zderad, 1988). Nurses acknowledge in theory that clients deserve more than merely technical care, but in practice nursing takes the path of least resistance, allowing itself to be readily lured by advances in medical science and more technically intricate curing (Spicker & Gadow, 1980). The marginalization of nursing's core values has been sustained by the discipline's failing to claim its own identity and seceding to bureaucratic and technocratic roles imposed by more emphatic political interests. In failing to anticipate or appreciate the social dynamics with which it is both suppressed and continuously reshaped for public consumption, nursing became the embodiment of the very feminine stereotypes and roles ascribed to it. Yet the situation is not inevitable, for humanistic education need not be inimical to rational, technical, and scientific training (Freire, 1970; Paterson & Zderad, 1988) and can be empowering—even in the face of domination by the elite (Kelner, 2000). However, since "therapeutic technology" includes the machines' overseers and technicians as well as the machines themselves, unresolved issues of values continue to threaten nursing's present and future.

Nursing's educational compromises are often obscured by the fact that it is possible to be technically expert without being either a professional (Benner, Tanner & Chesla, 1992; Benner, Hooper-Kyriakidis & Stannard, 1999; Watson, 1988) or broadly educated. Science-based empirical nursing describes, explains, predicts, and acts, while ethical nursing is about transcending techniques to focus on duty, rights, obligations, and moral imperatives (Benner, 2000; Benner, Tanner & Chesla, 1996). Esthetic knowing can tie science-based empirical nursing and ethical nursing together through personal understanding of self in relation to others in a caring presence (Smith, 1992). Yet little is known about how the representing, interpreting, and envisioning (Smith, 1992) required for such an esthetic process—that is, the imagining needed for caring— is efficaciously taught. Student vulnerability to the strains of value conflict has not been much attended to in nursing's pedagogies (Hughes, 1992). The need for development and evaluation of research-based paradigms and pedagogical practices for use at the core of nursing education is tremendous, but, given that most scholarship pertaining to alternative pedagogies stems from schools of education and remains more academic than applied, nurse educators are rarely stimulated to seriously consider the pedagogic assumptions and commitments embedded in their teaching (Ironside, 2001). And there is little funding available for those inclined to do ongoing study of nursing's pedagogies.

As if conspiring with the apprenticeship model into which early nursing education was compressed, nursing's pedagogies fell into patterns that negated many of its alleged ideals by treating students as objects; standardizing mechanical and industrial language across nursing roles; focusing on cognitive-technical techniques; valuing competency over caring and compassion; restricting teaching-learning to behavioral objectives, factual information, and methods; reinforcing dependence roles for teachers and learners; separating doing from knowing and from being; tolerating accreditation practices that conflict with nursing's moral and ethical beliefs, educational philosophies, and basic goals; and emphasizing entry into practice and credentials rather than helping students learn how to engage in social, moral, and scientific practices (Watson, 1988). That these pursuits have been widely and uncritically accepted is not surprising, given both nursing's pedagogical origins and its heavy investment in the Tylerian model of education.

During the mid-1940s, the influence of Dewey's powerful educational ideas gave way to the more readily articulated and researched aspects of empirical behaviorism. The Tylerian curriculum, which came along in 1950, fit well with the goal of the mass production of efficient nurses in its commitment to measurable behavioral objectives and formulated curriculum development (Bevis & Watson, 1989). In the manner common to the fragmentation of oppressed groups, and in line with the written-in-stone configuration of most of nursing's pedagogies, nursing developed a blurred, tri-part curricula over time. There was the legitimate curriculum agreed upon by faculty and written into formalized plans, a secondary curriculum that allowed some recognition of insights and creativity but was at odds with the predominately displayed behavioral objectives, and a hidden curriculum of subtle socialization that blended itself insidiously into teaching, prioritizing and interacting— and from which students learned to think and feel as nurses (Bevis, 1988).

As adopted by nursing, Tyler's educational model was technical and based on assumptions that the information would be applicable in clinical practice, and that such information must be acquired. It was also assumed under this model as applied to nursing that experience was necessary in each specialty area, while there was greater skepticism about the more amorphous aspects of teaching and learning, such as dialogue, empowerment, positive interaction between teachers and learners, and situated learning that encourages the "making of meaning" (Diekelmann, 1988, p. 153). Tylerian education also brought home the oppression of women with the formulation of so-called "critical" thinking, which was widely instituted despite the discipline's fundamentally limited educational breadth and depth. Nursing's core value of caring would fit well with humanistic education involving transformation and the lessening of oppression (Greenleaf, 1988), but nursing school culture, organization, leadership, and pedagogy (Epp & Watkinson, 1997) as well as the discipline's steadfast rationality rendered the learning environment anything but emancipatory (Habermas, 1979).

Issues deeply embedded in nursing's past and present have often rendered educational policy, transmission of knowledge, and management of learning confused and suspect (Diekelmann & Rather, 1993). With time, gaps between value and fact and between theory and practice became normative (Hiraki, 1992). Pedagogical agendas increasingly fostered development of competitive and outcome-related theories (Burbules & Torres, 2000; Lingard, 2000), while tension between a broad-based liberal education and a criteria-based behavioristic education created a conflict for educators unable to satisfactorily serve multiple masters. Few openly resisted including the arts or humanities in nursing education, but how they were to be used to benefit nurses and patients was vague in the otherwise largely scientifically precise pedagogical context. The social sciences, watered down to token levels, fared little better.

Certainly one part of nursing's rational commodity dilemma, which is reflected in the disciplines dominant pedagogies, is the context of caring. Many of nursing's contemporary ideologies and pedagogies claim to be about health, but remain wedded to the idea of complimenting medicine through paradigms deeply committed to specific scientific convictions (Botha, 1989) focused on ill-health, treatment and cure, not care. Having been thus claimed by external ideologies that pervade and persuade its thinking and comportment, it is not surprising that nursing's own core has been in large part relegated to its tattered fringes. Theory from practical rationality can be dialectically related to social action and praxis, but those often require more autonomy, depth, and introspection than nursing has had to invest. With pedagogies presenting nursing process in ways that separate it from the social institutions that shape everyday living, contexts (such as political or economic conditions) that influence its application are ignored (Hiraki, 1992).

Straddling a rational-objectivist model of education oriented toward medical science *and* a neglected philosophical, moral context of health and human caring (Watson, 1988), nursing seems to be sitting by, overwhelmed, while other disciplines find alternatives to the services once associated with it. The cacophony of nursing perspectives instigates self-doubt, uncertainty, and ambiguity (Gunby, Chally, Dorman, Grams, Kosowski, & Pless, 1991). Historically, educational opportunities for women as teachers advanced a mere step ahead of their students. Women filled a need formed by the creation of public schools, increasing population, and the westward growth of the nation, although the United States was even then committed to public education that was as cheap as possible (Kliebard, 1999). Given the cultural inclination to define both nursing and teaching as natural functions of women, it was one of nursing's successes that its leaders prevented nurse training from being totally subsumed into service programs (Flood, 1981). With the prolonged lack of differentiation between student and graduate nurse, it was a triumph to be able to establish the distinction between them—and the distinction between them and subsidiary workers. Nursing also won the struggle to increase cognitive content in nursing education. However, ultimately, nursing education was commodified, reflecting the long-term movement in tertiary education toward science and technology, which emphasizes academic capitalism at the expense of basic education, fundamental research, and scholarship. Fluidity of money, people, ideas, and goods characterizes global life today, while neo-conservative fundamentalism underwrites a shift from liberal to vocational education, from intrinsic to instrumental values of education, and from qualitative to quantitative measures of success (Blackmore, 2000). The impact of the ideology of the dollar sign as the bottom line has been profound. Nursing has been no less affected than the rest of society.

The discipline has a strong history of participation in community and public health, and that participation constitutes the most professional, autonomous, and academic of its orientations and practice settings (though most nurses still work in hospitals). Even there, where the industrialization of domestic labor has resulted in low status, low pay positions (Harding, 1980), nurses are discouraged from committing their work to direct patient care when their training and backgrounds have prepared them for tasks only indirectly related to patients, such as case coordination and utilization review (Joel, 1988). It is predicted that the paid labor market in health-related fields in the future will be dominated by low-paying, repetitive work with the most job growth occurring at the level of orderlies and aides (Apple, 2000). Growing numbers of chronically ill and frail elderly clients require more lower-level activities in therapeutic plans, while cost-consciousness promotes more and better use of the lesser skills of subsidiary personnel, volunteers, patients, and families (Joel, 1988). As health and medical care in the United States has shifted to clinic-based settings located in communities, nursing personnel in many cases have been replaced by auxiliary medical and other non-nursing staff.

The exigencies of cost containment may not appear directly related to the nature versus nurture debate. However, the assumption that women are naturally suited to caring has inhibited nursing's professionalization in that it is presumed that since caring comes naturally to women, they don't need to be paid for doing it. In a culture virtually obsessed with personal autonomy, a large proportion of adult Americans do volunteer work (Wuthnow, 1991). Caring participation in charitable activity, and the satisfaction derived from giving motivated by love or compassion, sets up obstacles in the perennial quest for fair and full remuneration for nursing services, as well as to achieving the needed synthesis of humanistic and scientific aspects of health (Paterson & Zderad, 1988; Spicker & Gadow, 1980). In nursing's failing to *own* its essential purposes and goals, outside pressures brought about their inversion. Narrowing investment in nursing faculty development, forced by market economics, led to valuing advanced practice clinicians (who tend to be clinically expert professionals, but not necessarily broadly educated) over academic expertise and experience. While ongoing development of nursing's clinical orientation is essential, its tenuous identification with academic scholarship is further compromised when only faculty with terminal degrees in nursing are considered appropriate role models and teachers.

In recent decades, some nurse educators have acknowledged and acted on the conflicts generated by nursing's pedagogical fixation with rationality and technical knowledge. Clinical teaching is developing alternative learning styles and taking place in new settings (Woolley & Costello, 1988). Yet, concerns loom as the nursing discipline increasingly focuses on advanced practice without facilitating the transition from a clinically oriented education to an academic orientation for those nurses who proceed to doctoral studies in their field, and without extensive efforts to bring nursing into meaningful conversation with other health professions. It is through informed use of language that pedagogical transformation can occur. Where is there evidence of nursing's abandoning passive, reactive silence in favor of a meaningful, educated voice? The liberated voice should be especially clear in helping new nurses to care about and act upon nursing's social position. It also stands to reason that nursing's doctorally prepared faculty and leadership should be the most articulate in this discourse. However, in circular fashion, conventional pedagogies perpetuate conventional doctorates and faculty. Developing the pedagogic literacy of nursing faculty remains an unmet priority (Ironside, 2001). Can faculty whose preparation has been more professional and applied than academic and theory-oriented, and who in many cases have never made the transition from clinical thinking to scholarship (for increasingly complex technical thinking and writing does not necessarily make it more scholarly), and who may little understand the social dynamics shaping their discipline, provide future nurses with the education that they will need to commit themselves to sustaining nursing?

Nursing's Hegemonic Pedagogical Dilemma

It is not accidental that things are the way they are.
Greenleaf, 1988, p. 121

For the past several millennia in Western societies, subjugation involving domination and exclusion has been premised on ideas derived from the social system of patriarchy (Bartky, 1979; Lerner, 1977). Within that context, women have a "double consciousness" a sense of themselves as being both central and marginal, essential and "other" (Lerner, 1997). Nursing developed in a time and place in which there was enormous change, but society still maintained an emphasis on women's roles as primarily submissive. A nurse trying to practice as a caring and humane professional in the present system finds herself or himself enmeshed in institutionalized remnants of paternalism and technological determinism. Practitioners of biomedicine routinely encounter therapeutic environments in which goals of healing have been systematically replaced by narrow technical objectives and the rules of efficiency and cost-effectiveness in bureaucratic medicine (Kleinman, 1995). No doubt physicians are as frustrated by this state of affairs as nurses are, but although both may experience a sapping of the vitality that generates therapeutic power and facilitates healing, the former are more often allowed to displace anger onto the latter than vice versa.

To some extent, every historical time is unsettling. Culture is never static; there is inevitably both change in it and resistance to such change. There are always good teachers who empower their students and who are empowered by them (Robinson, 1994), just as there are always potential new hegemonies that might come along to complicate the widespread use of empowering practices. But ignoring power relations amounts to reinforcing them to the benefit of those holding the power

(Lerner, 1997). Nursing has done relatively little to alter those relatic
Since negotiating is an activity essential for the mutual adjustment ui
both nurse and institution (Flood, 1981), much of the adjusting has been
done by nurses. That is, compromise is essential to the regulation of the
relationship between nurse and institution, but because nurses in general lack the power to negotiate, they do most of the compromising.
Politicians relaxed after passage of the Nineteenth Amendment when
they found that women could not deliver a bloc vote and that there were
few leaders who were interested in political careers; the "ladies" were
more interested in reform than politics (Flexner, 1975). Since then, the
presence of large numbers of women in any field has usually been interpreted as an argument for *not bothering* to organize it. Nurses generally
accept hospital-imposed dictates that unionization and grass-roots organizing are nonprofessional, which helps maintain nursing's second
class status. Despite a century of nursing history, there is no research
linking nursing's social status to its political nonchalance (Roberts,
2000). Yet the study of structural violence in the form of "social structures characterized by poverty and steep grades of social inequality"
(Farmer, 2002, p. 54) and, in particular, of horizontal violence are
deeply relevant to nursing where, in both clinical practice and nursing
education, nursing managers and administrators frequently flex their
traditionally hierarchical muscle rather than support nurses and nursing.

Nurses rarely talk about these things in public (Roberts, 2000), although the extent to which people effectively contend with such patterns of socially accepted (institutionalized) discrimination is occasionally studied and debated, and their forecasts pessimistic (Farmer, 2002).
Social and economic rights tend to be neglected within the realm of the
human rights community as unrealistic or impractical. That functional
abandonment is the result of hegemony, which generates resistance to
the cost that change would incur upon the more powerful players. However, it is widely agreed that social transformation, and even grasping
the consequences of structural violence, depends on understanding both
the structure and the process of change (Farmer, 2002). Nursing, overall, has been more sensitive to the plight of other groups (e.g., Barbee,
1993) than cognizant of its own situation. At the same time, the discipline's potential for advocacy of both self and others has been sorely
compromised by its quest for acceptance in the medical sphere (Hoff,
1994; Jackson, 1994). Nursing's seduction by the medical paradigm has

left it subject to victimization by the same professionalism elitism that it advocates against for its clientele.

Nursing's history and pedagogies have fostered a tradition of limited confidence in the discipline's own possibilities. Neither interested nor educated in the potency of politics, nursing internalized a "second class" status reinforced by hegemonic aspects of its relationships with the medical establishment and hospital labor practices, as well as by its compromised pedagogies. Nursing's lack of agency throughout much of its own history is reflected in the sociopolitical status that continues to inhibit its progress. For instance, nurse practice acts have typically legally supported the dependent and patronizing system of medical control over nursing functions. The line between medical and nursing activities with respect to diagnosing and treating is vague but at the same time the position is perpetuated by nurses in proscribing the parameters of their practice to ensure that nurses do not function independently. The initial premise that medicine and nursing would not compete evolved into a tacit conviction that nursing could or should not compete with medicine, so it has remained an extension or complement of biomedicine and not a substitute for it. Although nursing's image may be less negative now than at times in the past, the discipline's diverse credentials and roles have complicated its identity (Aroskar, 1980).

There are striking parallels between nursing's history in the United States and the process of colonialism in which the subordinate entity is separate and different, as defined and delimited by the colonizer, which in this comparison refers to the medical establishment. Normal, adaptive change by the colonized group (nursing) is impaired by the colonizer, and then the colonized suffers further with inadequate educational systems (Memmi, 1965). Eventual assimilation of the colonized into the colonizer is the price paid by the colonized for narrowing the gap between themselves and the colonizer in terms of prestige, power, and wealth. Advanced practice nursing might do well to heed the risks of becoming too much like medicine, for marginalization resumes when emulation precludes full acceptance by or identification with the colonizer.

Nursing's pedagogies are not the only ones challenged to find meaning in the United States today, where society has allowed the corporate subculture to reduce the priorities of education to the pragmatics of market demand for compliant, spectorial, and passive consumers. Yet conventional pedagogies continue to predominate in the production of nurses at both undergraduate and graduate levels. Oriented toward outcomes and problem-solving, conventional pedagogies emphasize efficient and effective provision and amassing of fact-laden information (Ironside, 2001). The same standardization of education that facilitates teaching and evaluating large groups reinforces modernist assumptions of a single truth, set of ethics, approach to rationality, and body of knowledge. There is little room in such a paradigm for multiple interpretations or the making of new meanings. Learning is institutionalized along with the entrenched values of authority, objectivity, mastery, and rationality. Despite claims to educate democratically, in actuality, the model is a colonial one designed to train in ways that devalue the intellectual dimensions of teaching and learning (Chomsky, 2000). The dominant aspects of society see the social order being domesticated for its own self-preservation. At the same time, at the local level students are rewarded for adjusting to models of learning that minimize understanding of the complexity of relations among phenomena (Chomsky, 2000). It is notable that the manufacture of colonial culture routinely involves engaging society's intellectuals and knowledge through technology (Goonathilake, 1982). Curative biomedicine, which replaces alternative ways of healing with legitimized, medicocentric systems, is viewed as one of the strongest media for colonization (Bulhan, 1985; Fanon, 1967; Goonathilake, 1982).

Administrative complicity in educational colonization is based on the classic assumption that authority is a suitable foundation for pedagogy. This gives teachers and administrators permission to subjugate learning, to use force to achieve adherence, and to systematically silence the non-adherent (Epp & Watkinson, 1997). Few nursing pedagogies have moved entirely beyond the common techniques of power in pedagogy (Gore, 1998). Authentic reflectivity, independent thought, and true critical thinking are sacrificed to techniques, procedures, and instrumental skills banks (Chomsky, 2000). Meanwhile, nursing practice is more complex than it used to be and entry level curricula are ever more challenged to establish an ethos of accountability for practice (Joel, 1988). At the same time, economic pressures tempt nursing programs to employ narrowly prepared faculty despite the fact that nursing desperately needs teachers who are educated beyond the exigencies of clinical practice.

More has been written about oppressed group behavior in nurses than about the discipline's liberation from oppression. Given the need to challenge inequality of power, coalition building is a major goal. The sense of inferiority that plagues nursing also interferes with efforts to empower itself to take control of its own destiny (Roberts, 2000). Subordinate groups learn to disparage themselves because the dominant group is able to set the norms for what is valued (Freire, 1971). Such "second class status" is internalized, resulting in more structural violence *within* than between groups. Success in the oppressed group then depends on looking and acting as much as possible like the dominant group (Roberts, 2000). Such is the case when nursing administrators are seen as joining the powerful (medical and hospital administrators and physicians) or when nurse practitioners or other advance practice clinicians are denigrated as "mini-docs." The internalized status differential is directly pertinent to nursing pedagogies because it is education that reinforces the belief that the dominant group's characteristics and abilities are the more important (Freire, 1971; Roberts, 2000). Over time, reflecting their hegemonic legacy, both groups come to believe that the status discrepancies are based on substantive differences and reflect a natural state of affairs—and the history of the hierarchy is lost to obscurity (Roberts, 2000).

Freire's stages for liberation from oppression hold promise and potential for nursing, should the discipline choose to go through them. The first, logically, is understanding the cycle and exposing the myths that maintain the hierarchy. This, unfortunately, is something rarely accomplished. The values of nursing are scarcely recognizable in patient care because the values of medicine and the medical model have been internalized by nurses as more appropriate (Roberts, 2000). To change this, nursing must gain autonomy and do away with its negative self-image. That would be difficult but possible if the discipline confronted its oppressed status as well as the strong pattern of passive acceptance of that status in it. Nursing would then need to be reinterpreted in terms of the social position of and discrimination against women (Roberts, 2000). The next phases involve learning how to work equitably with the dominant group *while* supporting nursing's own identity, and then learning to resolve the conflict between the old (negative) and new (more positive) identities. The final aspect of the transformative process involves the commitment needed to put the new perspective and identity into action (praxis). This achieved, nurses could then form closer and more empathic emotional ties with other nurses and eventually integrate their new, truly positive nursing identities into their lives (Roberts, 2000).

Effective pedagogy can be a form of resistance and progressive political action (Weiler, 1998). However, the predominant pedagogical model, which emphasizes the banking of pre-digested information, is so ineluctably institutionalized that faculty attempting to turn away from it find themselves challenged by bureaucratic practices and student expectations (Epp & Watkinson, 1997). Given the age-old commitment to deterministic, teacher-proof curricula (Carlson & Apple, 1998), "critical pedagogy" can find itself unwelcome in the educational encounter, although in recent years it has been gaining appreciation in some innovative settings. Generally, however, staying in education entails concession to codified bodies of knowledge about specific fields of inquiry and official information that provides quick fixes and claims to be authoritative and objective, with the expectation being that the student need only consume and learn them (Apple, 1993; Carlson & Apple, 1998). These rationalistic patterns are so much a part of contemporary culture that students come to nursing wanting and expecting to learn only marketable skills. So it is that in nursing, assimilation with medicine is desired and encouraged even as it is maligned. Normalization is dependent upon the punitive power of "othering" (Foucault, 1979) and, unlike many colonized societies, nursing retains a more idealized than real memory of things being different (Bartky, 1979). However, history is also about the healing of self representation. History can give voice to experience and give it new form that influences how future generations experience their lives. History does matter.

Nursing's More-of-the-Same (New Old) Versus Transformative Pedagogic Dialectic

The place where we are is in the middle of no way out.
Maly, 2001

In preparing nurses to be useful and employable, nursing's pedagogies have historically failed to address the issue of *how* to educate while preparing quality "products" for institutional use and *how* to prepare educated nurses as full professionals (Watson, 1988). It would be unfair to criticize pedagogical approaches and applications for being narrow if, in reality, nursing and nursing education *choose* to prioritize technical training and the discipline neither respects nor expects broader perspectives. It seems, however, that the situation is one more of unconsidered drift than choice. There has been little exploration of how the broader contexts provided by liberal education affect nurses and nursing practice (Hagerty & Early, 1992). Moving beyond the Tylerian model requires motivating students to be responsible for their own learning agenda, acknowledging the different contributions of training and education, and emboldening faculty development. The feasibility of basic nursing's doing this while being committed to an increasingly complex generalist curriculum remains inadequately critiqued.

Nursing's pedagogies have not remained wholly unchallenged. For example, nurse educators recognized and acted on a need to give up the destructive assumptions of biological determinism (Munhall, 1988), although relatively few acknowledge the damage done by ignoring the social implications of such ideologies. Many acknowledge the dominant pedagogical model as only one option, but relatively few have genuinely explored realistic alternatives. Similarly, it is widely affirmed that scientific skill and technological proficiency are insufficient for quality nursing, yet the awareness leaves a void with no consensus on how to fill it. It is widely acknowledged that new nursing curricula and contexts must realistically deal with ethically and politically complex technologies and clinical judgments (Aroskar, 1988; Rieger, 2000; White, 2000), but again there is no consensus about how best to accommodate such demands. Many educators cling to the idea that nursing education needs a humanitarian paradigm to encourage caring as a moral ideal and to integrate philosophical theories of human caring, health, and healing (Watson, 1988), but its applicability often seems elusive. Various approaches and methods have been suggested for the transformation of nursing education and practice, but their feasibility and effectiveness are clouded by their generally untested theoretical properties. Strategies for implementation have also been proposed (for example, Valiga & Bruderle, 1997), but little research has been done. That is due in part to the unavailability of funding for research in nursing education, but it also speaks to nursing's somewhat ambivalent relationships with both research and the perplexities of teaching and learning. The development and implementation of newer teaching methods shaped by critical, feminist, postmodern, and phenomenological approaches require teachers with academic backgrounds in such approaches who are motivated to put these teaching/learning methods to the test.

Meanwhile, the pressures experienced by faculty to teach for clinical application and to stay current and marketable in those areas, the limitations of perspectives imposed by practices that denigrate nonnursing influences and outside points of view, and faculty preparation that is often more clinical than scholarly in focus (as well as grounded in conventional nursing pedagogies) call into question the level of curricular literacy available for meaningful transformation. Ironside (2001) provides a scholarly summary of five pedagogic approaches widely used in schooling, teaching, and learning in nursing. Most used is the conventional approach already described. Emphasizing cognitive gain, skill acquisition, expert teachers, large student-teacher ratios, and contrived learning situations, conventional pedagogies are teacher and content driven and monocultural in their assumption that nursing has one set of objectives and that learning merely adds more material to presumed preexisting, standardized foundational skills and abilities.

In contrast to conventional educational approaches, alternative pedagogies have emerged in the quest for educational reform. Interpretive in nature, these models reject the absolutism of universal knowledge and values for more contextualized and relativistic explications that are grounded in real life experience and that acknowledge differences in terms of culture, perception, and interpretation. In recent years, critical social theory has influenced alternative education with its foci on empowerment, community building, social action, and the collective good. Power is centered in learners through rational dialogue (Ironside, 2001). Other alternative pedagogic approaches to nursing education include a mélange of feminist philosophies, with teachers and students partnered in personal transactions involving full participation—that is, praxis (Hernández, 1997). There is recognition of a need for language that takes up the issues of differences, bias, privilege, and oppression in the context of teaching and learning, although the focus on gender tends to overshadow other aspects of diversity (Hernández, 1997; Ironside, 2001).

Postmodernism is a collective term for rejection of universal, hegemonic perspectives in favor of multivocality (Rose, 1992). Its primary themes include the deconstruction of meta or grand narratives of education and the construction of fluid, contextualized, historic, discursive, and relativistic knowledge (Ironside, 2001). The production of meaning and theoretical perspectives of knowledge involve the fragmenting of traditional teacher and student roles. Postmodern teaching and learning models tend to be more theoretical than practical and may be limited in their commitment to relativism. However, a particularly powerful pedagogical combination involves the use of critical and postmodern theory together to analyze discourse for power differentials and to engage actively in emancipatory struggles (Hall, 1999). While postmodernism is sometimes viewed as foisting chaos on the disciplined order of healthcare, other alternatives founded on phenomenologic approaches have gained momentum either in lieu of or in combination with conventional educational approaches. Phenomenologic models focus on storied dialogue, everyday life experiences, understanding, and meaning, and issues of co-participation and partnership among learners and teachers (Ironside, 2001). Teaching and learning, which involve the understanding and exploration of experiences common to both teachers and learners, are local, site-specific and highly contextual.

In additional attempts to remedy nursing's educational problems, Moccia (1988) advocates pointing nursing education in the direction of social responsibility and political action. Matteson (1995), with others, emphasizes community and neighborhood-based learning places and models. The possibilities are myriad, but tend to lose vigor when faced with proscriptive accreditation regulations and highly formulated national examination and state licensure requirements. Transcending behavioristic and instrumentalist approaches in nursing education requires decisiveness about the selection and sequencing of the knowledge that nurses need to practice, and the role of experience in nursing education (Diekelmann, 1988). Whatever the strategies implemented, real changes in nursing pedagogy are possible only if extant curricular and instructional alternatives are sincerely explored (Diekelmann, 1988). At the same time, there is a need to protect students against educational paradigms for which they may be unprepared (or which may leave them unprepared) or that graduates find impede collaborative practice. Transformation of the traditional curricula is sometimes idealized as a transition from dualistic thinking with its authoritative, either/or approach to critical thinking to a contextualized knowledge befitting a relativistic world. Yet, given the pragmatics of nursing practice, its pedagogical tendencies toward concreteness, and the exigencies of public education, that would be a hard-won transformation. In reality, to practice, nurse graduates must be creative and willing to take risks, which was not possible under traditional pedagogies that instilled a fear of failure, assumed a single correct response, and did little to encourage examining interrelationships among phenomena encountered in quotidian nursing practice (Valiga, 1988).

In the plethora of educational critiques and ongoing reformulations in nursing, only Narrative Pedagogy, a phenomenologic approach committed to overcoming the teacher-centeredness of conventional education by creating a place for new partnerships and communities, has been research-based in its development and put into actual well evaluated practice (Diekelmann, 2001; Ironside, 2001). Diekelmann calls for a critical, feminist, and phenomenological pedagogy that uses narrative to explicate teachers' practices and students' experiences, as well as to communicate effectively about caring. Used in conjunction with conventional approaches, Narrative Pedagogy simply moves the pedagogical mirrors to include the social interaction of both teachers and learners so experience becomes part of the discourse of education and is "open to being re-imagined within a broad sociohistorical, geopolitical, and cultural framework that underscores the complexity and situatedness of places, relationships, and practices" (Hernández, 1997, p. xi).

Through more than a decade of research with both teachers and learners, Diekelmann (1991, 1992, 1993, 2001), the creator of Narrative Pedagogy, has elicited a set of "Concernful Practices of Schooling Learning Teaching" that articulate the shared and common experiences that *really matter* in education. Those practices (gathering; creating places; assembling; staying; caring; interpreting; presencing; preserving reading, writing, thinking, and dialogue; and questioning [Diekelmann, 2001]) reflect views and values from across the alternative educational philosophies, in addition to those of conventional education. The center of attention is the converging conversations that create space and possibilities, and responses and understandings, that often do not occur in conventional education. Providing entry into a way of life that involves seeing, talking, and writing in ways open to new understandings and experiences (Hernández, 1997; Kleinman, 1995), Narrative Pedagogy promises a new understanding of the ontology of "nurse."

Truly transformative pedagogies in nursing education ought to build on past achievements while rejecting nursing's historical shortcomings (National League for Nursing, 1988). Such change requires teacher preparation that prevents the perpetuation of teaching as one has been taught. Rather than remaining burdened by rationalistic content, authoritarian restraints, and behaviorist models of objectives and functions, nursing would come to understand and *own* caring through education unified in the deepest of actual human ways of being and by meeting real peoples' real needs. Moreover, nursing would engage in meaningful conversation with other health disciplines and be able to critically assess learning in a world of discontinuity and multiplicity (McCarthy & Dimityriades, 2000). A development of a sense of agency and responsibility for what happens in client interactions is in no way automatic, particularly when nurses are invested in accomplishing multiple, complex, and competing tasks (Benner, Tanner, & Chesla, 1992). For effective practice, nurses must develop a sense of agency that allows them to recognize in an experientially based way issues that are relevant and meaningful in changing situations, and that allows them to achieve a level of expertise through which they are able to grasp the practical significance of situations (Benner, Tanner, & Chesla, 1992, 1996). Currently, in practice among the diverse populations that characterize the United States today, nurses typically are unprepared to recognize what is important to their clients; the burden generally falls on clients to clarify and protect the values they consider meaningful (Hiraki, 1992).

Nursing has been better at spinning pedagogical rhetoric than making good pedagogy happen. If the discipline were authentically distinguished by a philosophy of advocacy rather than by its functions, that advocacy would obviate the maternalism that, in nursing, replaces the paternalism that pervades American culture and society. Both dynamics intend a good for the other, but often violate that other's wishes and autonomy in the matter. The possibility of the good being determined by (rather than imposed on) the less powerful group is obviated (Gadow, 1980). In sum, the advocate role entails assisting in authentic decision making and goes beyond consumer protection. Historically, nursing curricula have been repetitive and its pedagogies more willing to rearrange content than to make substantive changes. Only three major shifts in nursing's pedagogies have played substantial parts in nursing education in the United States. After early-seventeenth-century religious responses to caring in Europe, there was the founding of modern nursing in the United States. in the 1860s with its focus on moral behavior and comportment. In 1917, publication of a Standard Curriculum for

Schools of Nursing optimized the standardization of state requirements for training. Finally Tyler's approach to curriculum development, which emerged in the 1950s, was unreservedly embraced (Bevis, 1988).

Any further major curricular change is yet to come, but to be workable it (or they) will have to require that nursing make its pedagogies more congruent with its philosophies of practice and research and will have to distinguish more clearly between training and education, as well as among types of learning (Bevis, 1988). To date, Diekelmann's is the only new pedagogy developed from sound educational tenets that has been implemented and evaluated for nursing practice (Diekelmann, 1991, 1992, 1993, 2001). Transformative nursing pedagogies would also recognize and support teachers becoming expert learners, affording them the space to analyze, critique, and recognize insights from multiple perspectives, as well as to identify and evaluate assumptions. Such a pedagogy would recognize representation of diverse experiences as a significant issue (including, for instance, the terms in which teacher and curriculum address students) and would, most likely, use all available methods to inquire into the nature of health-related (in the broadest sense) phenomena. It would project in informed ways from knowns to unknowns, engage in praxis that brings together theory, research, and practice and reduces tension between clinical and academic emphases, learn to appreciate how meanings of curriculum items get produced and interpreted, evaluate contextualized wholes, find meanings in experiences, ideas, and paradigms, and strategize in mindfully aware ways.

Multiculturalism, a logical extension of any ethics that takes into account differing realities (Kleinman, 1995), could be integrated throughout nursing pedagogies as part of its inclusive philosophy. Biases would be explicated and critiqued, with involvement in social movements advocated at all levels. Nursing's intervention in the dynamics of social conflict would be kindled by refutation of gendered, racialized, and class-based interpretations of the curricula by students and teachers at the local level (Burbules & Torres, 2000). Given the need for pedagogies flexible enough to prepare nurses for practice in a nearly infinite repertoire of sites and contexts, it stands to reason that the positive valuing of multiple ways of knowing would be part of that preparedness.

In summary, nursing has survived for more than a century, but its future is predicated on the ability to transform its pedagogies to create and own a true discipline of nursing, and to avert claims by medical, technical, or other rationalizations. The cultural positioning of both teachers and students will need to be recognized as important to developing strategies for change that will shape what counts as knowledge and is valued as practice, and that will encourage an understanding of continuities and discontinuities within and between categories (Carlson & Apple, 1998). Today's pedagogical challenges are increasingly about how to achieve flexibility and adaptability, how to develop learning strategies for coexistence with diverse others and in multifarious spaces, and how to help form and support a sense of identity that can sustain multiple contexts of affiliation (Burbules & Torres, 2000). These are not agendas that an apathetic, fragmented, and oppressed group can achieve. The question of how nursing came to be as it is now is superseded by "to what extent can nursing build on its past and present to actively reclaim and recreate its pedagogies for preparing students as nurses who can deal with the realities of status differentials and claim and own nursing practice?" Nursing has roots, no matter to what extent it chooses to heed or ignore them; now it needs to shape strong and confident wings (Mead, 1972). Put another way, if nursing means to survive, its days of feigning ignorance of the impact of class and gender dynamics on the shaping of women's and nurses' options must end. Nursing must learn to look directly into the mirror and to see the realities there. Having mirrors that reflect only each other do little to inform the need for change.

Note

1. On two occasions, admittedly some years apart, Nancy Diekelmann, Ph.D., Helen Denne Schulte Professor at the University of Wisconsin–Madison School of Nursing, asked me this question. When I could not answer it to my satisfaction, she challenged me to do so. This essay is dedicated to Nancy and her catalytic yen for deeper understandings.

References

Allen, D. (1987). Critical social theory as a model for analyzing ethic issues in family and community health. *Family and Community Health, 10*(1), 63–72.

Althen, G. (1988). *American ways: A guide for foreigners in the United States.* Yarmouth, ME: Intercultural Press.

American Nurses Association. (1965). *Educational preparation for nurses.* Washington, D. C.: American Nurses' Association.

Apple, M. W. (1988). *Teachers and texts: A political economy of class and gender relations in education*. New York: Routledge.

Apple, M. W. (1993). *Official knowledge: Democratic education in a conservative age*. New York: Routledge.

Apple, M. W. (1999). Between neoliberalism and neoconservatism: Education and conservatism in a global context. In N. C. Burbules & C. A. Torres (Eds.), *Globalization and education: Critical perspectives*. New York: Routledge.

Apple, R. D. (Ed.). (1992). *Women, health, and medicine in America: A historical handbook*. New Brunswick, NJ: Rutgers University Press.

Arendt, H. (1958). *The human condition*. Chicago: University of Chicago Press.

Aroskar, M. A. (1980). The fractured image: The public stereotype of nursing and the nurse. In S. F. Spicker & S. Gadow, (Eds.)., *Nursing: Images and ideals: Opening dialogue with the humanities*. New York: Springer.

Aroskar, M. A. (1988). Curriculum revolution: A bioethical mandate for change. In *Curriculum revolution: Mandate for change*. New York: National League for Nursing Press.

Ashley, J. A. (1976). *Hospitals, paternalism, and the role of the nurse*. New York: Teachers College Press.

Barbee, E. L. (1993). Racism in U. S. nursing. *Medical Anthropology Quarterly, 7*(4), 346–362.

Bartky, S. L. (1979). On psychological oppression. In S. Bishop, & M. Weinzweig (Eds.), *Philosophy and women*. Belmont, CA: Wadsworth Publishing.

Bastable, S. B. (1979). *Recruitment of students into basic nursing education programs in the United States, 1893–1949: An historical survey*. Unpublished doctoral dissertation. Ann Arbor, MI: University Microfilms International.

Baxandall, R., Gordon, L., & Reverby, S. (1976). *America's working women*. New York: Random House.

Bednash, G. (2000). The decreasing supply of registered nurses: Inevitable future or call to action? *Journal of the American Medical Association, 283*(22), 2985–2987.

Benhabib, S., & Cornell, D. (1987). Introduction. In S. Benhabib & D. Cornell (Eds.), *Feminism as critique: On the politics of gender*. Minneapolis: University of Minnesota Press.

Benner, P. (2000). The wisdom of our practice: Thoughts on the art and intangibility of caring practice. *American Journal of Nursing, 100*(10), 99–105.

Benner, P., Hooper-Kyriakidis, P., & Stannard, D. (1999). *Clinical wisdom and interventions in critical care: A thinking-in-action approach*. Philadelphia: W. B. Saunders.

Benner, P., Tanner, C. A., & Chesla, C. A. (1992). From beginner to expert: Gaining a differentiated clinical world in critical care nursing. *Advances in Nursing Science, 14*(3), 13–28.

Benner, P., Tanner, C. A., & Chesla, C. A. (1996). *Expertise in nursing practice: Caring, clinical judgment, and ethics*. New York: Springer Publishing.

Berkhofer, R. F., Jr. (1995). *Beyond the great story: History as text and discourse*. Cambridge, MA: Belknap.

Bevis, E. O. (1988). New directions for a new age. In *Curriculum revolution: Mandate for change*. New York: National League for Nursing Press.

Bevis, E. O., & Watson, J. (1989). *Toward a caring curriculum: A new pedagogy for nursing*. New York: National League for Nursing (Pub. no. 15–2278).

Bishop, W. J., & Goldie, S. (1962). *A bio-bibliography of Florence Nightingale*. London: Dawsons of Pall Mall for the International Council of Nurses.

144 KAVANAGH

Blackmore, J. (1999). Globalization: A useful concept for feminists rethinking theory and strategies in education? In N. C. Burbules & C. A. Torres (Eds.), *Globalization and education: Critical perspectives*. New York: Routledge.

Botha, M. E. (1989). Theory development in perspective: The role of conceptual frameworks and models in theory development. *Journal of Advanced Nursing, 14*(1), 49–55.

Brown, E. L. (1948). *Nursing for the future: A report prepared for the national nursing council*. New York: Russell Sage Foundation.

Brown, P. J. (Ed.). (1998). *Understanding and applying medical anthropology*. London: Mayfield Publishing.

Brownlee, W. E., & Brownlee, M. M. (1976). *Women in the American economy: A documentary history, 1675 to 1929*. New Haven, CT: Yale University Press.

Bulhan, H. A. (1985). *Frantz Fanon and the psychology of oppression*. New York: Plenum.

Burbules, N. C., & Torres, C. A. (1999). Globalization and education: An introduction. In N. C. Burbules & C. A. Torres (Eds.), *Globalization and education: Critical perspectives*. New York: Routledge.

Bush, M. A., & Kjervik, D. K. (1979). The nurse's self-image. In D. K. Kjervik & I. M. Martinson (Eds.), *Women in stress: A nursing perspective*. New York: Appleton-Century-Crofts.

Cades, H. (1930). *Jobs for girls*. New York: Harcourt, Brace.

Candy, B. H. (1979). Florence Nightingale: Woman with a vision. In D. K. Kjervik & I. M. Martinson (Eds.), *Women in stress: A nursing perspective*. New York: Appleton-Century-Crofts.

Carlson, D., & Apple, M. W. (Eds.). (1998). *Power/knowledge/pedagogy: The meaning of democratic education in unsettling times*. Boulder, CO: Westview Press.

Carnegie, M. E. (1986). *The path we tread: Blacks in nursing, 1854–1984*. Philadelphia: Lippincott.

Carroll, B. A. (Ed.). (1976). *Liberating women's history: Theoretical and critical essays*. Urbana: University of Illinois Press.

Césaire, A. (1972). *Discourse on colonialism* (J. Pinkham, Trans.). New York: Monthly Review Press.

Chinn, P. L., & Wheeler, C. E. (1985). Feminism and nursing. *Nursing Outlook, 33*(2), 74–77.

Chomsky, N. (2000). *Chomsky on MisEducation*. (D. Macedo. Ed.). Lanham, MD: Rowman & Littlefield.

Cimprich, B. (1992). A theoretical perspective on attention and patient education. *Advances in Nursing Science, 14*(3), 39–51.

Cleland, V. (1971). Sex discrimination: Nursing's most pervasive problem. *American Journal of Nursing, 71*(8), 1542–1547.

Coburn, D., & Willis, E. (2000). The medical profession: Knowledge, power and autonomy. In G. L. Albrecht, R. Fitzpatrick, & S. C. Scrimshaw (Eds.), *Handbook of social studies in health and medicine*. Thousand Oaks, CA: Sage.

Cohen, M. N. (1998). Culture, not race, explains human diversity. *Chronicle of Higher Education*, April 17, B4–B5.

Comaroff, J. L., & Comaroff, J. (1992). *Ethnography and the historical imagination*. Boulder, CO: Westview.

Commission on Hospital Care. (1947). *Hospital care in the United States: A study of the function of the general hospital, its role in the care of all types of illness, and* the conduct of activities related to patient service: With recommendations for its extension and integration for more adequate care of the American public. New York: Commonwealth Fund.

Committee on Curriculum of the National League of Nursing Education. (1937). *A curriculum guide for schools of nursing.* New York: National League of Nursing Education.

Committee on the Grading of Nursing Schools. (1931). *First grading: School control.* New York: Committee on the Grading of Nursing Schools.

Connolly, C. (2000). The TB preventorium. *American Journal of Nursing, 100*(10), 62–65.

Conrad, P., & Kern, R. (Eds.). (1994). *The sociology of health and illness: Critical perspectives* (4th ed). New York: St. Martin's.

Cott, N. F. (Ed.). (1972). *Roots of bitterness: Documents of the social history of American women.* New York: Dutton.

Cott, N. F., & Pleck, E. H. (Eds.). (1979). *A heritage of her own: Toward a new social history of American women.* New York: Simon & Schuster.

Cunningham, M. P. (2000). Breaking the mold: The many legacies of nurses in progressive movements. *American Journal of Nursing, 100*(10), 121–136.

Darwin, C. (1958). *The origin of species: By means of natural selection or the preservation of favoured races in the struggle for life.* New York: Penguin Books. (Original work published in 1859.)

David, B. A. (2000). Nursing's gender politics: Reformulating the footnotes. *Advances in Nursing Science, 23*(1), 83–93.

Dawley, K. (2000, October). The campaign to eliminate the midwife. *American Journal of Nursing, 100*(10), 50–56.

Deloria, V., Jr. (1985). *American Indian policy in the twentieth century.* Norman: University of Oklahoma Press.

Denzin, N. K. (1997). *Interpretive ethnography: Ethnographic practices for the 21st century.* Thousand Oaks, CA: Sage.

De Tornyay, R. (1991). Creating community among nurse educators. In *Curriculum revolution: Community building and activism.* New York: National League for Nursing Press.

Devitt, N. (1979). The statistical case for the elimination of the midwife: Fact versus prejudice, 1890–1935. *Women and Health, 4*(1, 2), Part 1. 81–96. Part 2. 169–186.

Diekelmann, N. L. (1988). Curriculum revolution: A theoretical and philosophical mandate for change. In *Curriculum revolution: Mandate for change.* New York: National League for Nursing Press.

Diekelmann, N. L. (1991). The emancipatory power of the narrative. In *Curriculum revolution: Community building and activism.* New York: National League for Nursing Press.

Diekelmann, N. L. (1992). Learning-as-testing: A Heideggerian hermeneutical analysis of the lived experiences of students and teachers in nursing. *Advances in Nursing Science, 14*(3), 72–83.

Diekelmann, N. L. (2001). Narrative pedagogy: Heideggerian hermeneutical analyses of lived experiences of students, teachers, and clinicians. *Advances in Nursing Science, 23*(3), 53–71.

Diekelmann, N. L., & Rather, M. L. (Eds.). (1993). *Transforming RN education: Dialogue and debate.* New York: National League for Nursing Press. Pub. No. 14–2511.

Dock, L. L. (1903). The duty of this society in public work. *Proceedings of the American Society of Superintendents of Training Schools*.

Dolan, J. A. (1963). 1893–1912: Fusing the past for future action. In *"Three score years and ten": 1893–1963*. New York: National League for Nursing Press.

Donaldson, L. E. (1992). *Decolonizing feminisms: Race, gender and empire building*. Chapel Hill: University of North Carolina Press.

Dorland, W. A. N. (1908). *The sphere of the trained nurse*. (Address given at the Philadelphia School of Nursing, 27 May).

Dossey, B. M., Keegan, L., & Guzzetta, C. E. (2000). *Holistic nursing: A handbook for practice*. Gaithersburg, MD: Aspen.

Douglas, A. (1977). *The feminization of American culture*. New York: A. A. Knopf.

Dreves, K. D. (1963). 1933–1952: Measuring up. In *"Three score years and ten": 1893–1963*. New York: National League for Nursing Press.

Ehrenreich, B., & English, D. (1978). *For her own good: 150 years of the experts' advice to women*. Garden City, NY: Anchor Press.

Elder, Frances. (1958). Why nurses don't stay put. *RN, 21*, 67.

Epp, J. R., & Watkinson, A. M. (Eds.). (1997). *Systemic violence in education: Promise broken*. Albany: State University of New York Press.

Etienne, M., & Leacock, E. (Eds.). (1980). *Women and colonization: Anthropological perspectives*. New York: Praeger.

Ewing, N. H. (1935). The head nurse as executive: An analysis of ward responsibility. *Trained Nurse and Hospital Review, 94*, 224–227.

Fanon, F. (1967). *Black skin, white masks* (C. L. Markmann, Trans.). New York: Grove Press.

Farmer, P. (2002). Structural violence and the assault on human rights. *Anthropology News, 43*(1), 54–55.

Finkler, K. (2000). *Experiencing the new genetics: Family and kinship on the medical frontier*. Philadelphia: University of Pennsylvania Press.

Flexner, E. (1975). *Century of struggle: The women's rights movement in the United States*. (Rev. Ed.). Cambridge, MA: Belknap.

Flood, M. E. (1981). *The troubling expedient: General staff nursing in United States hospitals in the 1930s, a means to institutional, educational, and personal ends*. Unpublished PhD dissertation, University of California, Berkeley (Education). Ann Arbor, MI: University Microfilms International.

Foucault, M. (1979). *Discipline and punish: The birth of the prison* (A. Sheridan, Trans.). New York: Vintage. (Original French work published in 1975.)

Fowler, W. W. (1886). *Woman on the American frontier: A valuable and authentic history of the heroism, adventures, privations, captivities, trials, and noble lives and deaths of the "Pioneer mothers of the republic."* Hartford, CT: S. S. Scranton.

Frank, G. (2000). *Venus on wheels: Two decades of dialogue on disability, biography, and being female in America*. Berkeley: University of California Press.

Franklin, B. M. (Ed.). (2000). *Curriculum and consequence: Herbert M. Kliebard and the promise of schooling*. New York: Teachers College Press.

Fraser, N. (1987). What's critical about critical theory? The case of Habermas and gender. In S. Benhabib & D. Cornell (Eds.), *Feminism as critique: On the politics of gender*. Minneapolis: University of Minnesota Press.

Fredrickson, G. M. (2000). *The comparative imagination: On the history of racism, nationalism, and social movements*. Berkeley: University of California Press.

Freire, P. (1970). *Pedagogy of the oppressed* (M. B. Ramos, Trans.). New York: Herder & Herder.

Freire, P. (1982). *Education for critical consciousness* (M. B. Ramos, Trans.). New York: Continuum.

Gadow, S. (1980). Existential advocacy: Philosophical foundation of nursing. In S. F. Spicker & S. Gadow (Eds.), *Nursing: Images and ideals: Opening dialogue with the humanities*. New York: Springer.

Gamarnikow, E. (1978). Sexual division of labour: The case of nursing. In A. Kuhn & A. M. Wolpe (Eds.), *Feminism and materialism: Women and modes of production*. London: Routledge and Kegan Paul.

Garrison, D. (1979). *Apostles of culture: The public librarian and American society, 1876–1920*. New York: Free Press.

Giele, J. Z. (1995). *Two paths to women's equality: Temperance, suffrage, and the origins of modern feminism*. New York: Twayne Publishers.

Giddens, A. (1982). *Profiles and critiques in social theory*. Berkeley: University of California Press.

Glass, L. K., & Brand, K. P. (1979). The progress of women and nursing: Parallel or divergent. In D. K. Kjervik & I. M. Martinson (Eds.), *Women in stress: A nursing perspective*. New York: Appleton-Century-Crofts.

Goffman, E. (1961). *Asylums: Essays on the social situation of mental patients and other inmates*. Garden City, NY: Doubleday.

Goldmark, J. (1923). *Nursing and nursing education in the United States*. New York: Macmillan.

Good, M. J. D. (1998). *American medicine: The quest for competence*. Berkeley: University of California Press.

Goonathilake, S. (1982). *Crippled minds: An exploration into colonial culture*. Delhi, India: Vikas.

Goostray, S. (1963). 1913–1932: Emerging values. In *"Three score years and ten": 1893–1963*. New York: National League for Nursing Press.

Gordon, A. D., & Buhle, M. J. (1976). Sex and class in colonial and nineteenth-century America. In B. A. Carroll (Ed.), *Liberating women's history: Theoretical and critical essays*. Urbana: University of Illinois Press.

Gore, J. M. (1998). On the limits of empowerment through critical and feminist pedagogies. In D. Carlson & M. W. Apple (Eds.). *Power/knowledge/pedagogy: The meaning of democratic education in unsettling times*. Boulder, CO: Westview Press.

Graduates versus students. (1933). *American Journal of Nursing, 33*(3), 473–481.

Greenleaf, N. P. (1988). Historical and economic perspectives on the nursing labor force. In *Curriculum revolution: Mandate for change*. New York: National League for Nursing Press.

Grey, G. G. (1931). The past, present, and future of nursing education. *Modern Hospital, 36*(1), 124–128.

Griffin, G. J., & Griffin, H. J. K. (Eds.). (1965). *Jensen's history and trends of professional nursing* (5th edition). Saint Louis. MO: Mosby.

Grimké, A. E. (1838). *Letters to Catherine E. Beecher*. Boston: Lodge.

Gunby, S. S., Chally, P., Dorman, R. E., Grams, K. M., Kosowski, M. M., & Pless, B. S. (1991). Alice in Wonderland: A metaphor for professional nursing education. In *Curriculum revolution: Community building and activism*. New York: National League for Nursing Press.

Habermas, J. (1975). *Legitimation crisis* (T. McCarthy, Trans.). Boston: Beacon Press. (Original German work published in 1973.)

Habermas, J. (1979). *Communication and the evolution of society* (T. McCarthy, Trans.). Boston: Beacon Press. (Original German work published in 1976.)

Hagerty, B. M. K., & Early, S. L. (1992). The influence of liberal education on professional nursing practice: A proposed model. *Advances in Nursing Science, 14*(3), 29–38.

Hall, J. M. (1999). Marginalization revisited: Critical, postmodern, and liberation perspectives. *Advances in Nursing Science, 22*(2), 88–102.

Ham, W. (1932). The case study method of nursing. *Pacific Coast Journal of Nursing, 28*(3), 84–85.

Hamilton, P. M. (1992). *Realities of contemporary nursing*. (No location): Addison Wesley Nursing.

Harding, S. (1980). Value-laden technologies and the politics of nursing. In S. F. Spicker & S. Gadow (Eds.), *Nursing: Images and ideals: Opening dialogue with the humanities*. New York: Springer.

Harding, S. (1987). *Feminism and methodology: Social science issues*. Bloomington: Indiana University Press.

Harris, B. J, (1978). *Beyond her sphere: Women and the professions in American history*. Westport, CT: Greenwood.

Haugh, K. H. (2000). "Nursing by default:" The evolution of floor nursing, 1900–1965. *Windows in Time (Center for Nursing Historical Inquiry), 8*(2), 5–7.

Hawke, M. (2001). Declining enrollment: An educator's view. *Nursing Spectrum, 5*(16), 24.

Hedin, B. (1986). A study of oppressed group behavior in nurses. *Image: Journal of Nursing Scholarship, 18*(2), 53–57.

Heidegger, M. (1971). *On the way to language* (P. D. Hertz, Trans.). New York: Harper & Row.

Heidegger, M. (1999). *Contributions to philosophy: From enowning*.(P. Emad & K. Maly, Trans.). Bloomington: Indiana University Press. (Original German work published in 1989.)

Hernández, A. (1997). *Pedagogy, democracy, and feminism: Rethinking the public sphere*. Albany: State University of New York Press.

Hiestand, W. C. (2000, October). Think different: Inventions and innovations by nurses, 1850 to 1950. *American Journal of Nursing, 100*(10), 72–77.

Hine, D. C. (1989). *Black women in white: Racial conflict and cooperation in the nursing profession, 1890–1950*. Bloomington: Indiana University Press.

Hiraki, A. (1992). Tradition, rationality, and power in introductory nursing textbooks: A critical hermeneutics study. *Advances in Nursing Science, 14*(3), 1–12.

Hoff, L. A. (1994). Comments on race, gender, and class bias in nursing. *Medical Anthropology Quarterly, 8*(1), 96–99.

Hogeland, R. W. (Ed.) (1973). *Women and womanhood in America*. Lexington, MA: Heath.

Hosler, K. (2001, December 22). Senate, House seeking cure for nation's nurse shortage. *The [Baltimore] Sun*, p. 3A.

Hrebinak, L. G. (1974, September). Job technology, supervision, and work-group structure. *Administrative Science Quarterly, 19*, 395–410.

Hughes, L. (1992). Faculty-student interactions and the student-perceived climate for caring. *Advances in Nursing Science, 14*(3), 60–71.

Ironside, P. M. (2001). Creating a research base for nursing education: An interpretive review of conventional, critical, feminist, postmodern, and phenomenologic pedagogies. *Advances in Nursing Science, 23*(3), 72–87.

Jackson, E. M. (1993). Whiting-out difference: Why U. S. nursing research fails black families. *Medical Anthropology Quarterly, 7*(4), 363–385.

Jackson, E. M. (1994). Commentary and reply: Whiting-out difference: Why U.S. nursing research fails black families. *Medical Anthropology Quarterly, 8*(2), 219–220.

Jensen, D. M. (1942). *Principles and practice of ward teaching*. Saint Louis: Mosby.

Joel, L. A. (1988). The impact of DRGs on basic nursing education and curriculum implications. In *Curriculum revolution: Mandate for change*. New York: National League for Nursing Press.

Joralemon, D. (1999). *Exploring medical anthropology*. Boston: Allyn and Bacon.

Kalisch, P. A., & Kalisch, B. J. (1995). *The advance of American nursing* (3rd edition). Philadelphia: Lippincott.

Katz, M. S., Noddings, N., & Strike, K. A. (Eds.). (1999). *Justice and caring: The search for common ground in education*. New York: Teachers College, Columbia University.

Kaufman, M. (1976). *American medical education: The formative years, 1765–1910*. Westport, CT: Greenwood Press.

Kavanagh, K. H. (1988). The cost of caring: Nursing on a psychiatric intensive care unit. *Human Organization, 47*(3), pp. 242–251.

Kavanagh, K. H. (1991). Invisibility and selective avoidance: Gender and ethnicity in psychiatry staff interaction. *Culture, Medicine, & Psychiatry, 15*(2, June), pp. 245–274.

Kavanagh, K. H. (1995). Collaboration and diversity in technology transfer. In T. E. Backer, S. L. David, & G. Soucy (Eds.), *Reviewing the behavioral science knowledge base on technology transfer* (pp. 42–64). U.S. Department of Health and Human Services, PHS, NIH. Rockville, MD: National Institute on Drug Abuse, NIDA Research Monograph 155.

Kavanagh, K. H., & Kennedy, P. H. (1992). *Promoting cultural diversity: Strategies for health care professionals*. CA: Sage.

Kavanagh, K. H., Kennedy, P. H., Kohler, H. R., & Rasin, J. H. (1993). Exploring the experience of African American students in a school of nursing. *Journal of Nursing Education, 32*(6), 273–275.

Keeling, A., & Ramos, M. C. (1995). The role of nursing history in preparing nursing for the future. *Nursing and Health Care, 16*, 30–34.

Keller, P. (1932, July). The doctor's viewpoint toward the education of the nurse. *Bulletin of the American Hospital Association, 6*, 111–19.

Kelly, L. Y. (1985). *Dimensions of professional nursing* (5th edition). New York: Macmillan.

Kelner, D. (1999). Globalization and the new social movements: Lessons for critical theory and pedagogy (pp. 300–322). In N. C. Burbules & C. A. Torres (Eds.), *Globalization and education: Critical perspectives*. New York: Routledge.

Kleinman, A. (1995). *Writing at the margin: Discourse between anthropology and medicine*. Berkeley: University of California Press.

Kliebard, H. M. (1999). *Schooled to work: Vocationalism and the American curriculum, 1876–1946*. New York: Teachers College Press.

Kottack, C. P. (1999). *Mirror for humanity: A concise introduction to cultural anthropology*. Boston: McGraw-Hill College.

Kreisberg, S. (1992). *Transforming power: Domination, empowerment, and education*. Albany: State University of New York.

Lawler, J. (1993). *Behind the screens: Nursing, somology, and the problem of the body*. Redwood City, CA: Benjamin/Cummings.

Lerner, G. (1977). *The female experience: An American documentary*. Indianapolis, IN: Bobbs-Merrill.

Lerner, G. (1997). *Why history matters: Life and thought*. New York: Oxford University Press.

Levi-Strauss, C. (1963). *Structural anthropology*. New York: Basic Books.

Lewenson, S. B. (1996). *Taking charge: Nursing, suffrage, and feminism in America, 1873–1920*. New York: NLN Press, Publication no. 14-6843.

Lewin, E. (1977). Feminist ideology and the meaning of work: The case of nursing. *Catalyst, 10–11*, 78–103.

Lingard, B. (1999). "It is and it isn't": Vernacular globalization, educational policy, and restructuring. In N. C. Burbules & C. A. Torres (Eds.), *Globalization and education: Critical perspectives*. New York: Routledge.

Litoff, J. B. (1992). Midwives and history. In R. D. Apple (Ed.), *Women, health, and medicine in America: A historical handbook*. New Brunswick, NJ: Rutgers University Press.

Lobove, R. (1965). *The professional altruist: The emergence of social work as a career, 1880–1930*. Cambridge: Harvard University Press.

Lundh, U., Soder, M., & Waeness, K. (1988). Nursing theories: A critical view. *Image, 20*(1), 36–40.

MacEachern, M. T. (1940). *Hospital organization and management* (2nd edition). Chicago: Physicians Record Company.

Maly, K. (2001, June 28). Paraphrasing M. Heidegger, *On the way to language*. Nursing Institute for Heideggerian Hermeneutical Studies, University of Wisconsin–Madison, 26–30 June.

Margolis, M. L. (1984). *Mothers and such: Views of American women and why they changed*. Berkeley: University of California Press.

Marks, J. (1994). Black, white, other. *Natural History*. December, 32–35.

Matteson, P. S. (Ed.). (1995). *Teaching nursing in the neighborhoods: The Northeastern University model*. New York: Springer.

McCarthy, C., & Dimityriades, G. (2000). Globalizing pedagogies: Power, resentment, and the re-narration of difference.

McClain, C. S. (Ed.). (1989). *Women as healers: Cross-cultural perspectives*. New Brunswick, NJ: Rutgers University Press.

Mead, M. (1972). *Blackberry winter: My earlier years*. New York: Simon and Schuster.

Meeting of the Board of Directors. (1938). *American Journal of Nursing, 38*(3), 324–331.

Melosh, B. (1982). *"The physician's hand": Work culture and conflict in American nursing*. Philadelphia: Temple University Press.

Memmi, A. (1965). *The colonizer and the colonized*. New York: Orion Press.

Mill, J. S. (1869). Sexism as inequality. *The subjection of women*. London: Shepard.

Moccia, P. (1988). Curriculum revolution: An agenda for change. In *Curriculum revolution: Mandate for change*. New York: National League for Nursing Press.

Morrow, R. A., & Torres, C. A. (1999). The state, globalization, and educational policy. In N. C. Burbules & C. A. Torres (Eds.), *Globalization and education: Critical perspectives*. New York: Routledge.

Munhall, P. L. (1988). Curriculum revolution: A social mandate for change. In *Curriculum revolution: Mandate for change*. New York: National League for Nursing Press.

Myers, S. L. (1982). *Westering women and the frontier experience, 1800–1915.* Albuquerque: University of New Mexico Press.

National Commission for the Study of Nursing and Nursing Education. (1970). Summary, report and recommendations. *American Journal of Nursing, 70*(3), 270–289.

National League for Nursing. (1988). Preface. *Curriculum revolution: Mandate for change.* New York: National League for Nursing Press.

Navarro, V. (1976). *Medicine under capitalism.* New York: Prodist.

Nicholson, L. (1987). Feminism and Marx: Integrating kinship with the economic. In S. Benhabib & D. Cornell (Eds.), *Feminism as critique: On the politics of gender.* Minneapolis: University of Minnesota Press.

Nicholson, L. (1990). Introduction. In L. Nicholson (Ed.), *Feminism/Postmodernism.* New York: Routledge.

Nightingale, F. (1858). *Notes on matters affecting the health, efficiency, and hospital administration of the British Army, founded chiefly on the experience of the late war, presented by request to the Secretary of State of War.* London: Harrison and Sons.

Nightingale, F. (1859a). *A contribution to the sanitary history of the British Army during the late war with Russia.* London: Harrison and Sons.

Nightingale, F. (1859b). *Notes on hospitals.* London: John W. Parker and Sons.

Nightingale, F. (1859c). *Notes on nursing: What it is, and what it is not.* London: Harrison and Sons.

Norris, K. (1998). *The quotidian mysteries: Laundry, liturgy and "women's work."* New York: Paulist Press.

Oakley, A. (1974). *The sociology of housework.* Oxford, England: Martin Robertson.

Oakley, A. (1984). The importance of being a nurse. *Nursing Times.* December 12, 24–27.

Oates, L. (1938). Advanced professional curricula. *American Journal of Nursing, 38*(8), 909–916.

Parrillo, V. N. (1990). *Strangers to these shores: Race and ethnic relations in the United States.* New York: Macmillan.

Paterson, J. G., & Zderad, L. T. (1988). *Humanistic nursing.* New York: National League for Nursing. Pub. No. 41–2218.

Pavey, A. E. (1938). *The story of the growth of nursing.* London: Faber & Faber.

Peters, M. (1996). *Poststructuralism, politics and education.* Westport, CT: Bergin & Garvey.

Peters, M., Marshall, J., & Fitzsimons, P. (1999). Managerialism and educational policy in a global context: Foucault, neoliberalism, and the doctrine of self-management. (PP. 109–132). In N. C. Burbules & C. A. Torres (Eds.), *Globalization and education: Critical perspectives.* New York: Routledge.

Petry, L. (1937). Basic professional curricula in nursing leading to degrees. *American Journal of Nursing, 37*(2), 287–297.

Public School Instruction on Cooking. (Editorial) (1899). *Journal of the American Medical Association, 32*(9), p. 1183.

Richards, J. R. (1980). *The skeptical feminist: A philosophical enquiry.* London: Routledge & Kegan Paul.

Ricoeur, P. (1983). *Hermeneutics and the human sciences* (J. Thompson, Trans.). London, England: Cambridge University Press.

Rieger, P. (2000). The gene genies. *American Journal of Nursing, 100*(10), 87–90.

Roberts, M. (1937). Florence Nightingale as a nurse educator. *American Journal of Nursing, 37*(6), 775.

Roberts, M. M. (1954). *American nursing: History and interpretation*. New York: Macmillan Company.

Roberts, S. (1983). Oppressed group behavior: Implications for nursing. *Advances in Nursing Science, 5*(4), 21–30.

Roberts, S. J. (2000). Development of a positive professional identity: Liberating oneself from the oppressor within. *Advances in Nursing Science, 22*(4), 71–82.

Robinson, J. A. (1994). *The ethnography of empowerment: The transformative power of classroom interaction*. Washington, DC: Falmer Press.

Rose, M. A. (1992). *The post-modern and the post-industrial: A critical analysis*. Cambridge, England: Cambridge University Press.

Rossi, A. S. (Ed.). (1970). *Essays on sex equality: John Stuart Mill and Harriet Taylor Mill*. Chicago: University of Chicago Press.

Rothman, S. M. (1978). *Woman's proper place: A history of changing ideals and practices, 1870 to the present*. New York: Basic Books.

Sandercock, L. (Ed.). (1998). *Making the invisible visible: A multicultural planning history*. Berkeley: University of California Press.

Schmidt, D. B., & Schmidt, E. R. (1976). The invisible woman: The historian as professional magician. In B. A. Carroll (Ed.), *Liberating women's history: Theoretical and critical essays*. Urbana: University of Illinois Press.

Sellow, G. (1930). *A textbook of ward administration*. Philadelphia: Saunders.

Sklar, K. K., Schüler, A., and Strasser, S., (Eds.). (1998). *Social justice feminists in the United States and Germany: A dialogue in documents, 1885–1933*. Ithaca, NY: Cornell University Press.

Slaughter, S., & Leslie, L. (1997). *Academic capitalism: Politics, policies and the entrepreneurial university*. Baltimore: Johns Hopkins University Press.

Smith, M. J. (1992). Enhancing esthetic knowledge: A teaching strategy. *Advances in Nursing Science, 14*(3), 52–59.

Spicker, S. F. & Gadow, S., (Eds.). (1980). *Nursing: Images and ideals: Opening dialogue with the humanities*. New York: Springer.

Stewart, E. C., & Bennett, M. J. (1991). *American cultural patterns: A cross-cultural perspective*. Yarmouth, ME: Intercultural Press.

Stewart, I. M. (1936). Preparing nurses to meet the changing needs of society. *42nd Proceedings of the NLNE*. New York: National League for Nursing Education.

Stowe, H. B. (1981). *Uncle Tom's cabin, or life among the lowly* (A. Douglas, Ed.). Hammondsworth, U. K.: Penguin.

Street, A. (1992). *Inside nursing*. Albany: State University of New York Press.

Symonds, A. (1991). Angels and interfering busybodies: The social construction of two occupations. *Sociology of Health and Illness, 13*(1), 249–264.

Therese, Sr. M. (1936). Newer methods of teaching in schools of nursing. *Trained Nurse and Hospital Review, 97*, 457–460.

Thompson, J. (1987). Critical scholarship: The critique of domination in nursing. *Advances in Nursing Science, 10*(1), 27–38.

Tocqueville, A. de. (1969). *Democracy in America* (G. Lawrence, Ed. J. P. Mayer, Trans.). New York: Harper Perennial.

Tsosie, R. (2000). Changing women: The crosscurrents of American Indian feminine identity. In V. L. Ruiz & E. C. DuBois (Eds.), *Unequal sisters: A multicultural reader in U.S. women's history* (3rd edition). New York: Routledge.

Tulloch, G. (1989). *Mill and sexual equality*. Hertfordshire, U. K.: Harvester Wheatsheaf.

Union membership? No! (1930). *American Journal of Nursing, 38*(4), 573–574.

Universities and nursing education. (1934). *Trained Nurse and Hospital Review, 92,* 162.

Valiga, T. M. (1988). Curriculum outcomes and cognitive development: New perspectives for nursing education. In *Curriculum revolution: Mandate for change.* New York: National League for Nursing Press.

Valiga, T. M., & Bruderle, E. R. (1997). *Using the arts and humanities to teach nursing: A creative approach.* New York: Springer.

Vertinsky, P. A. (1994). *The eternally wounded woman: Women, doctors and exercise in the late nineteenth century.* Urbana: University of Illinois Press.

Vogel, M. (1980). *The invention of the modern hospital: Boston, 1870–1930.* Chicago: University of Chicago Press.

Watson, J. (1988). A case study: Curriculum in transition. In *Curriculum revolution: Mandate for change.* New York: National League for Nursing Press.

Wayland, M. M., McManus, R. L. M., & Faddis, M. O. (1944). (I. M. Stewart, Ed.). *The hospital head nurse: Junior executive and clinical instructor.* New York: Macmillan.

Weiler, K. (1998). Respondent: Pedagogy for an oppositional community. In D. Carlson & M. W. Apple, (Eds.). *Power/knowledge/pedagogy: The meaning of democratic education in unsettling times.* Boulder, CO: Westview Press.

Welter, B. (1966). The cult of true womanhood: 1820–1860. *American Quarterly, 18*(1), 151–174.

Wetzel, S. M. (1936, September). What's wrong with the nursing in our hospitals? *Trained Nurse and Hospital Review, 97,* 244–247.

White, G. B. (2000). What we may expect from ethics and the law. *American Journal of Nursing, 100*(10), 114–117.

Whyte, M. K. (1978). *The status of women in preindustrial societies.* Princeton, NJ: Princeton University Press.

Wilson, C. (1930). Character. *American Journal of Nursing, 30*(2), 278.

Woodham-Smith, C. B. F. (1951). *Florence Nightingale: 1820–1910.* New York: McGraw-Hill.

Woolley, A. S., & Costello, S. E. (1988). Innovations in clinical teaching. In *Curriculum revolution: Mandate for change.* New York: National League for Nursing Press.

Wuthnow, R. (1991). *Acts of compassion: Caring for others and helping ourselves.* Princeton, NJ: Princeton University Press.

3

Listening to Learn

Narrative Strategies and Interpretive Practices in Clinical Education

Melinda M. Swenson and Sharon L. Sims

Introduction

Clinical education in the health professions arises from a long tradition of lecture, demonstration, mentoring, apprenticeship, practice, memorization, repetition, and objective testing. The focus has been on content and the achievement of teacher-directed outcomes. This traditional model has worked well in the past, but is being challenged as the world of healthcare undergoes rapid and unpredictable change. No longer can the teacher lecture from last year's notes or use the same written exam semester after semester. The classroom instructor cannot stay current without constant attention to and direct experiential contact with the clinical world. One of the problems with traditional, content-driven education (in addition to the obvious one created when content exceeds the ability to keep up with it) is that it conflates content application with thinking. Indeed, any clinical curriculum driven by content alone is suspect by its very nature (Diekelmann & Diekelmann, 2000).

This article describes the experience of students (and teachers) in an innovative master's program in nursing, one that uses new pedagogies in a Narrative-Centered Curriculum (Swenson & Sims, 2000).[1] Our pedagogies focus on seeking, hearing, responding to, reflecting on, and interpreting clinical and personal stories of students, patients, preceptors, and teachers. We discuss the results of teaching and learning using a variety of narrative approaches, including reading and writing clinical

154

stories and case studies, listening to stories from patients and clinicians, and discussing and reflecting on how clinical stories can enhance and transform clinical practice. These pedagogical strategies, employed in a site-specific advanced practice nursing program, could be adapted and modified to use in any clinical discipline. We blend traditional techniques (classroom discussion, written assignments, preceptored clinical practice) and unconventional approaches (narrative, interpretive, and reflective strategies). The combined pedagogies use narrative thinking to call forth reflective listening in students, teachers, and clinicians, and result in learning situated in experience.

Educational and Philosophical Bases for the Curriculum

Schön refers to formalistic, traditional thinking in clinical practice as *technical rationalism* (1983, p. 50). He contrasts this concept with *knowing-in-action* and *reflection-in-action*, which are more effective in the unique and uncertain contexts so common in clinical situations. Knowledge of content does not require any particular attention or reflection unless one is concerned with simply acquiring more content, or doing more complex tasks, or doing more things at once. Teachers and clinicians know that content knowledge is not enough, yet cling to traditional pedagogies privileging content and procedural knowledge because these strategies are familiar and comfortable.

In this approach, we agree with Bateson (1994). Bateson approaches narrative not only as story, but as a powerful vehicle for vicarious experience and subsequent change. She writes: "Our species thinks in metaphors and learns through stories" (p. 11). Similarly, Coles (1990) proposes that viewing science as a series of narratives is revolutionary, and that stories are the origin of change in thinking and in skilled practices. Narratives are the connection between experience and interpretation.

As teachers, we are concerned with the discrepancy between our commitment to empirically grounded clinical practice and our preference for qualitative research. Our conviction is that nursing, as both an art and a science, is a holistic and integrated discipline that should not be compartmentalized into "quantitative" and "qualitative" components. We also believe that nursing and other human science disciplines are interpretive in nature, especially at the advanced practice level, because we focus on individual people and their unique experiences. If we expect clinicians to be mindful listeners and thoughtful practitioners, then the teaching and learning offered must also be interpretive in nature. The Narrative-Centered Curriculum[2] enables teachers to "put their minds where their hearts are" in the realm of teaching and learning and to use pedagogical approaches reflecting both a scientific and a phenomenological and experiential[3] view of the world of clinical practice. Bringing narratives into clinical education and practice may serve to improve the art of healthcare, while preserving critical aspects of empirical science.

Another foundation for our educational approaches lies in interpretive and narrative pedagogy. Diekelmann (2001) developed her new pedagogies to meet rapidly changing needs in clinical nursing. Narrative Pedagogy is not a single teaching or curricular strategy, but rather an approach that creates an opening for all kinds of teaching and learning to co-occur in classroom and clinical arenas. Narrative Pedagogy is a way of thinking about teaching and learning that grounds and enables all possibilities. The Narrative-Centered Curriculum encourages a gentle gestalt shift that both accommodates and challenges the way things are, and makes cognitive and emotional changes possible in teachers and learners.

We are also influenced by the American pragmatists John Dewey (1938), who emphasized that experience—personal and social—is the best teacher, and Richard Rorty (1999, p. 54), who proposed usefulness as the aim of inquiry. According to Dewey, experiences are always connected to other experiences and to the context in which they occur, and learning always takes place within the context of the experience. Because narratives communicate experience-in-context, we place them at the center of teaching and learning. The usefulness of experience-based practice, within a context of empirical evidence, is clear to us as we visit students, talk to clinicians, and work with preceptors. Polkinghorne (1988) ventures even further, suggesting that narrative is the base and basis for clinical work. He points out that "[practitioners] are concerned with people's stories: they work with case histories and use narrative explanations to understand why the people they work with behave the way they do" (p. x). Certainly this description sums up nurse practitioners' work with patients and families.

Professional Bases for the Curriculum

The Pew Health Professions Commission (1995) and other professional organizations, including the American Association of Colleges of

Table 3.1   NONPF (2002) Domains of Clinical Practice

Domain 1:	Managing Patient Health/Illness Status
	Health Promotion/Health Protection and Disease Prevention
	Managing Patient Illness
Domain 2:	The Nurse Practitioner-Patient Relationship
Domain 3:	The Teaching-Coaching Function
	Eliciting information
	Assisting patients
	Providing health information and counseling
	Negotiating plan of care
	Coaching the patient throughout the care experience
Domain 4:	Professional Role
	Developing and implementing role
	Directing care
	Providing leadership and advocacy
Domain 5:	Managing and Negotiating Health Care Delivery Systems
Domain 6:	Monitoring and Ensuring the Quality of Health Care Practices
Domain 7:	Cultural Competence (includes spiritual competencies)

Nursing (1996) and the National Organization of Nurse Practitioner Faculties (2000–2001), published recommendations for practice competencies of graduates required to meet the healthcare needs of the next century. These recommendations and guidelines form the basis for curriculum development in clinical education generally, and also are specific to advanced nursing practice. According to a study by Bellack, Graber, O'Neil, Musham, & Lancaster (1999), directors of nurse practitioner programs indicated the three most important curriculum topics identified by respondents were "primary care," "health promotion/disease prevention," and "effective patient-provider relationships and communication." The study found that barriers to change included curricula already overcrowded with content, and limited availability of clinical sites for preceptored practice. In addition, these authors found similar needs and barriers in the curricula of other health professions.

The National Organization of Nurse Practitioner Faculties (NONPF) developed core competencies for all nurse practitioners and specialty competencies for family nurse practitioners and four other areas (available online at *www.nonpf.org*). Competencies assist nursing faculty in curriculum development, provide guidelines for state boards of nursing, and help employers and third-party payers set expectations regarding nurse practitioner scope of practice. The competencies are based in eight domains of practice, first delineated by Brykczynski (1989) and later incorporated into *NONPF Curriculum Guidelines for Nurse Practitioner Programs* (1995).

Our Family Nurse Practitioner (FNP) program meets the Pew Commission recommendations and the NONPF competencies, with special emphasis on those areas considered most important: primary healthcare, health promotion, illness prevention, and patient-clinician communication. We use evidence-based practice (when effectiveness and efficiency are an issue) and practice-based learning (when more inductive issues are raised) in addition to narratives and stories. We wanted to use narrative to tie together these and other deductive and inductive and reflective approaches to keep open many paths to learning.

Conventional Clinical Education

In health professions education, teachers' own histories of learning influence the ways they teach and what they choose to evaluate. We tend to teach as we were taught, and most of us learned in traditional ways. This teaching was intended to be efficient, to be technologically sophisticated, to change behavior and encourage the memorization of content, and to be teacher-dominated. Barr & Tagg (1995) describe this kind of teaching as an instructional paradigm, where the following conditions prevail:

- Emphasis on content as the most important aspect of instruction, and acquisition of factual knowledge as the most important product of teaching and learning. The main purpose of classroom instruction is to convey content. Teachers are the expert interpreters—perhaps the only interpreters—of the content. The teacher is the classroom executive, who mediates between content and learners. Information is transferred from teacher to learner via lectures, teacher-directed seminars and discussions, and teacher-directed assignments.
- In the instructional paradigm, students are regarded as novices who are assumed to know little and are a homogeneous group. Personal experience is discounted as too unique and subjective.
- Reliance on testing and measurement as a guarantee of learning.
- Didactic/content aspects may be separated in time from clinical/experiential

aspects of education, sometimes by weeks or months. Different teachers may teach didactic and clinical courses, and communication between them may be sporadic.

Standard teaching approaches work well in many situations, and expert teachers know how to maneuver among a variety of strategies to promote knowledge acquisition by students. None of these approaches is wrong in and of itself. They have worked well for a long time in many disciplines. The emphasis on content, theory, evidence-based practice, problem-solving, and critical thinking is not misplaced and not without value. However, these strategies leave little room for new ways of thinking, new ways of conceptualizing problems, or new ways of interacting with students. Most traditional pedagogies allow no time at all for the previously unthought, the divergent, the tangential, or the unanticipated, and do not value these conditions as relevant sources of learning in clinical disciplines. We wanted to make room in the curriculum for all aspects of practice, including evidence-based clinical decision-making and problem-solving, technical skills, and explicit procedural knowledge. In addition, we wanted to find ways to enable students to learn how to be present with their patient, how to demonstrate listening practices, how to be reflective in their understanding of ethical issues and dilemmas, and how to preserve and celebrate curiosity and compassion.

Moving Toward a Narrative Approach

When we planned our FNP Master of Nursing Science (MSN) major at Indiana University School of Nursing, we were committed to building a program that took account of the NONPF Curriculum Guidelines (1995) and to meeting requirements of the various organizations offering national professional certification. The new major also had to conform to our school requirements: a maximum of 42 semester credits, including the 15 credits of required core courses for all MSN students. These courses included advanced practice roles, health policy, legal and ethical issues, nursing theory, and nursing research. Each student also was required to design and conduct an independent nursing research project. Within those boundaries, we developed our FNP major and admitted our first students in 1995.

Rather than an instructional paradigm, we employed a learning paradigm (Barr & Tagg, 1995) aimed toward education for understanding rather than instruction solely for content acquisition. Among other teaching strategies, we employed narrative pedagogical principles and approaches (Andrews et al., 2001; Ironside, 1999; Nehls, 1995). We built our pedagogy on the following principles:

- The Narrative-Centered Curriculum is a conscious, integrated, holistic approach to learning in nurse practitioner programs. It is not piecemeal, confined to just one course or to an isolated faculty member. We never want to present learning as content without context, an approach that promotes forgetting, inattention, and passivity. Rather, we concentrate on the whole of nursing practice as it presents itself in patient and family stories. Openness to all possibilities, including that of listening to stories and reflecting on them in practice, characterizes this curriculum.
- We discard the idea that all useful knowledge is cumulative and linear, and that we always must proceed from the simple to the complex. We see clinical knowledge as a series of nested and interactive frameworks, worked out by each individual learner with teacher guidance and coaching.
- We do not intend simply to transfer knowledge from teacher to student, but to create environments, opportunities, experiences, and openings that make possible students' discovery and construction of meaningful learning and that foster the ability to creatively imagine and solve problems they will encounter in practice.
- We are committed to developing connecting conversations among learners, teachers, families, patients, preceptors, and others.
- We believe that stories are an integral means of interpreting experience. Stories create a place with listening at the center.
- Telling stories, listening to stories, and reflecting on stories is an ideal way to make meaning of experience-based learning. This is what Frank (1995) would call "thinking with stories" (p. 158).

Using Narratives in the Curriculum

Why Narratives?

According to Polkinghorne (1988, p. 1), narratives are the primary form by which human experience is made meaningful. Narrative examples in clinical education may include patient stories of everyday and common experiences of health and illness, organized health histories and physical examinations, student and teacher stories of being new and being experienced in practice, and preceptor narratives of clinical decision making. All these sources are legitimate ways to ground and illustrate clinical experience. In clinical practice and in the classroom, experience teaches meaning, embodied knowing lives in experience, and human experience is grounded in the interpreted story.

Narratives compel us. A story recruits our willing attention. It leads us to reflect. A story tends to invite us to search for significance and to involve us personally, since our inclination is to seek the storyteller's meaning via our own interpretation. Stories are transformative. We may be touched, shaken, moved by a story. Stories teach us and we remember them. Stories are alive. Finally, stories provide a way to develop one's interpretive sense. One's response to a story is a measure of one's ability to make meaning (van Manen, 1991, p. 121). Stories are part of our everyday life, accessible and understandable, they allow—even celebrate—the meaning of experience. They provide useful information about what works and perhaps even more useful information about what does not work in clinical practice. The interpreted story is the foundation of new knowledge in the field. What stands out in every story is what is meaningful and useful to the listener and to the teller.

Reflecting on Narratives

Stories are necessary, but of course, in themselves not sufficient for safe clinical practice. The uninterpreted story provides only an interesting anecdote. Reflection, the process of thinking about and exploring issues, concerns, and clinical questions, especially when precipitated by listening to stories of lived experience, enables the clinician to incorporate changes permanently into practice. Clinicians also communicate modifications of practices to other providers via presentations and publications, thereby changing and improving the practice of the discipline. For patients, interpreting a story of illness can help illuminate the meaning of the particular illness and its impact on the person and the family. It can also help bring to light coping strategies, expectations and hopes, and deep concerns and fears. The purpose of the story and its interpretation is to make sense of the experience, to make it useful for practice, and to make it available to others. Listening to the story and attentively hearing its meaning benefits both the one cared for and the ones caring. This professional comportment provides support for patients and families as they seek to understand the meaning of health and illness and can be modeled and practiced during clinical education so that it becomes a part of the everyday life of the clinician.

When teachers welcome stories, they create openings for centered listening and reflective practices. The particular strategies we use are less important than the caring practices they engender in teachers and students. Components of the Narrative-Centered Curriculum that are narrative in orientation include patient histories, students' personal stories of caring, paradigm clinical cases, practice-based learning stories in class, stories from preceptors and faculty in class, and clinical discussions, both formal and informal. Our intent is to enable teachers and students to hear stories in whatever form they are presented, to make them aware of narratives in their clinical practice, and to enhance their ability to tell their own stories. Examples of uses of narrative in the curriculum are discussed in the following section.

Curricular Values and Components

We must emphasize that particular teaching strategies do not, by themselves, constitute a narrative pedagogy. Nor do narrative pedagogies make up the entire curriculum. We present specific approaches and techniques only as examples that show how storytelling, listening, and interpretation can occur together in classroom and clinical experiences to improve caring practice. We want to illustrate not that we use particular innovative teaching strategies, but that teachers in this program knowingly and deliberately create a learning environment where listening practices can emerge. We begin with the words themselves.

Words Matter

We want students to hear how language speaks, by helping them become more aware of and sensitive to the words they use in everyday practice. For example, in the physical assessment course, we encourage students to approach the patient history in a variety of ways, including through the use of traditional problem-oriented recording. They learn how to determine the reason for the patient's visit, including why the patient is being seen. Rather than calling this the "chief complaint," we use "chief concern" as a way of sensitizing students to the idea that the words used in the write-up of the history have an effect on how clinicians view patients. We use the term "history of the present issue" (rather than "history of the present illness," but still abbreviated HPI) and ask the patient to tell the story of their concern first, later filling in the details, including what the patient thinks might be the source of the trouble.

We pay attention to the actual words used as we discuss clinical issues because words have the power to create and maintain reality. Indeed, Socrates (cited in Fiumara, 1990, p. 148) suggests that listening bears human risks, leading him to the *maieutic* metaphor: that listening is the midwife to thinking and learning, that listening births thinking. For example, if students used words like "complains" and "denies" with reference to a patient, the patient could be seen as burdensome or as a person whose story ought to arouse suspicion.

Words do matter, and language conveys far more than words alone. Language speaks practice, and we must pay close attention to what we say and write. The words we choose indicate attitudes and beliefs, though we may be unaware of hidden meanings. By focusing on words used, we emphasize how the listener hears what is said and subsequently interprets meaning. For example, we encourage students to take a "health history" rather than a "medical history," choosing to use a term that encompasses a broader disciplinary boundary than medicine and that suggests that both health and illness are important components of a patient's history. To avoid sounding paternal and militaristic, students send lab "requests" rather than lab "orders." They avoid using "female" and "male" as nouns, and instead talk about women and men, children and teenagers. Students never refer to themselves as learning to be "midlevel providers" but rather as learning to be clinicians, a less hierarchical nomenclature.

Course Construction for Narrative Learning

Basic characteristics of our pedagogies are illustrated in our course syllabi. Our courses do not begin with a content outline. Students come to the program with such a wide variety of skills and such a range of knowledge that we think it impossible to predetermine specific content to meet these diverse educational needs. We also acknowledge the explosion of new knowledge in the discipline, and the rapid changes taking place in what we think we know. Using a modified version of practice-based learning (Barrows, 1994) in place of static, teacher-centered lectures, we bring real patients and families to each class and let them tell their stories of health and illness.[4] Students are not assigned reading prior to these classes in which they listen to these stories. Students and faculty listen and ask questions until they are satisfied that they have heard all that the family wants to tell them. We then identify the learning issues arising from the story. A learning issue is any question that must be answered to address the family's concerns or problems.

Each student chooses a set of learning issues they know little about and prepares a one-page summary regarding each to share with the class at the next meeting. These are not generic reports but are always tailored to the specific needs of the patient and family. When the story is fully analyzed and the reports presented to the group, the class develops a plan of care for the family. There may be some learning issues that remain unclear, or that students feel they need to know more about. These can be revisited, or students may request a consultation about specific elements of a learning issue unclear to them. Faculty or other experts may make a short presentation focused on the students' questions. Class discussions are lively conversations, with students, faculty, and clinical faculty all sharing their knowledge and expertise.

At the end of each clinical course, we organize the issues and situations discussed and summarize them in a topical content outline that is shared with students. In this way, content is not devalued, yet does not drive the learning. Learning issues are reconsidered in each course with new patient stories. For example, students learn about hypertension as it relates to women's health, and then again in their adult health course. They learn about asthma and its management in all three of their population-specific courses: women's health, adult health, and child health. In each instance, the issues are tailored to the needs of the particular patient and family. Students gain confidence in their ability to recall and apply knowledge and to add layers of new information to their knowledge base as they need it. All these practices model ways of thinking and learning about caring for families that are immediately and directly applicable in clinical practice.

Teachers in this curriculum hold in common our ideas about teaching, learning, and evaluation. We are willing to give up control over the content (but not the curriculum), willing to let patients teach our students, willing to stop being the center of the classroom, and willing to believe students are capable of evaluating their own learning. Classroom activities reflect faculty commitment to building meaningful connections among learners, teachers, families, and clinicians. The curriculum demonstrates that experience (and reflection on experience) is the best teacher, and that clinical stories and other narratives provide students with ways to reconstruct, reflect on, interpret, and learn from experience.

The Patient's History as Narrative

We introduce our narrative focus in the physical assessment course, where students learn to obtain and interpret patient histories and perform physical examinations. We emphasize the narrative value of the history, treating it as a story of the patient's experience with health or illness. Adler (1997, online) suggests that the history of an illness provided by the patient can be examined as narrative and experiential communication, and that the telling of it to a sensitive listener can be therapeutic in the telling and diagnostic in the listening. In addition, he cites the transformative nature of telling and listening to a history: "Because we grow up giving and getting each other's histories, we also know the satisfaction that can come from transforming the chaos of experience into a coherent narrative in the course of explaining that experience to someone else." Students have been accustomed to viewing health histories as information-gathering strategies, intended to produce a concise, organized catalog of the problem and its component parts. These health histories could be regarded as a template imposed on a patient's story in which the clinician picks and chooses to record only certain kinds of information, usually in the form of a list, ignoring other material that might take the form of a more vivid narrative account of the patient's life. However, if the patient history is regarded as an implicit narrative, it can serve as an index or outline of a more extended story, thereby increasing its meaning and usefulness for patient and clinician (White, 1981).

Bruner (1990) observes that:

In most interviews, we expect participants to answer our questions in the categorical form required in formal exchanges, rather than in the narratives of natural conversation . . . As interviewers, we typically interrupt our respondents when they break into stories, or in any case we do not code the stories: they do not fit our conventional categories. So the human Selves that emerge from our interviews become artificialized by our interviewing method. (p. 115)

In other words, it is easy for professionals to fall into the mode of listening only through the form and order of our questions. We are unable or unwilling to listen beyond our template of required information.

By hearing the patient's version of the illness narrative first, students are better able to determine the meaning of the illness to the patient and family. They also are in a position to focus on aspects of the illness that most worry the patient and are able to set priorities *with* the patient, rather than *for* the patient. Students learn to invite the story of a patient's concern, and then to plan with the patient to accomplish the patient's goals. A conversational approach, unhurried and undirected, builds rapport and shapes the relationship between clinician and patient, gives each time to think and consider what should be done, and leads the way to more connected communication that matures over time. In addition, this attention to the patient's story privileges the language of the person cared for, rather than the language of the clinician.

Personal Stories of Caring

Ricouer (1985) proposes that "Our own existence cannot be separated from the account we can give of ourselves. It is in telling our own stories that we give ourselves an identity" (p. 214). With the aim of developing an identity as nurse practitioners, we begin each clinical course with personal stories that help learners see who they are as nurses and nurse practitioners and that also acknowledge the personal identities of others in the classroom. Students write a titled story about a time they will never forget that relates directly to the course focus. For example, before starting the course "Primary Health Care of Children," students write a story about taking care of an ill child. Some write stories based in their nursing practice, some write about taking care of their own children, some write about being ill as children. Students read their story aloud to the class.

Students read the stories aloud because the shared experiences of telling the story and hearing the story are as important to the meaning as the content. Titling the story is a first step in interpretation and reflection. Titles help the student to distill the essence of the narrative and make that essence clear at the outset. Reading these stories and listening to them involves a basic trust. Students must trust that if they speak, the other members of the class will listen carefully, enabling them to interpret thoughtfully and respond accordingly. Listening to ourselves through speech or writing involves a hope and a belief that our thoughts are worth recording, and that they will be useful in learning and will not be exploited by others. Each story elicits commentary and appreciation from the other members of the class and builds personal connections between and among the learners and the teachers. Teachers also write and read their own stories as a means of illustrating that narratives, though unique, have meanings understandable by students. The stories, now common ground for the class, can be the source of discussion later in the course and in subsequent courses, each time enabling new meanings and new ways of thinking about patient care.

Paradigm Clinical Stories

Paradigm clinical stories are required assignments in each semester. These are memorable cases experienced by the student during the clinical rotation that he or she writes down. Paradigm case stories are written in traditional problem-oriented recording style or in a more narrative style. There are two additional steps. First, students describe what the experience taught them that they will never forget and how what they learned from this particular interaction with this particular patient will continue to inform their practice in the future. This reflective part of the paper is evaluated along with the paper. Students are provided with written guidelines for choosing a paradigm case story that help them focus on the learning experience and its meaning. A second deviation from tradition is that students write the patient educational plan verbatim, in the actual words they would use with the patient and family. This means they must adjust their vocabulary to meet the needs of the patient, must carefully select words that convey the meaning they desire, and must be careful to include salient features of the situation that take into account the cultural and personal values of the individual. The paradigm clinical story is presented partially as a narrative and partially as a "standard case write-up," with attention focused on both aspects.

Clinicians' Narratives

As often as possible, clinical faculty members attend the didactic sessions of a course. Having clinical faculty in the classroom provides yet another view of patient care that is grounded in the everyday practice of an expert. Many clinical faculty members are graduates of this program, and their stories carry extra credibility because they have been exposed to the same pedagogical strategies and have participated in the same learning activities as the current students. Clinical faculty sometimes have stories that provide conflicting views of how specific medications should be prescribed or how particular laboratory results should be interpreted; these discussions model the ways stories can be used to illustrate a point or negotiate a disagreement.

Self-Reflection and Self-Interpretation

Interpreting and reflecting, making meaning of stories in context, also illustrate listening practices. This process does not amount to naive relativism, in which any interpretation is as good as any other. Instead, we are focused on the best available interpretation that allows for the development of understanding. It is the act of self-reflection that makes interpretation possible. We have several ways of making this particular thinking practice visible to students.

Students write self-reflection statements at midterm and at the end of each of five clinical courses. Guidelines for these statements suggest looking at personal goals and objectives, but also encourage including stories that illustrate progress, demonstrate professional growth, or show meaningful learning. Students use these statements to convey fears, doubts, triumphs with respect to their learning, as well as challenges to it. Faculty members respond to the statements in writing, by commenting, encouraging, sharing insights, and pointing out successes. The student keeps the midterm evaluation and hands it in again at the end of the course, allowing him or her to reflect on progress since midsemester and make plans for future growth in the role. Students tell the stories, faculty listen and respond, and both offer interpretations of the significance and usefulness of the learning. We build a culture of listening by reflective practices.

Faculty members also offer their own self-reflective statements at the end of the program, explaining how the teaching was conceptualized, suggesting ways it might have been improved, and describing ways in which it succeeded. Teachers share their joys, concerns, worries, and triumphs. We offer this statement in an effort to make the teaching process more visible to the students, and as an instrument to model ongoing personal reflection in professional practice.

We wanted to study this narrative pedagogical approach to see how the active learning, reflective, narrative, and experiential components were experienced by the learner-in-the-world, and how this kind of learning might influence advanced practice nursing for our graduates. Our inquiry is described below.

Method

Our goal when we began this study was to examine the fir:
years of our new curriculum for the clinical education of advanced practice nurses. We wanted to understand how learning happened in our
narrative-centered curriculum, as well as what students learned. We
were interested in the quality of the interactions between and among
teachers and learners, and how learners were able to make meaning
from their schooling. We also wanted to know how graduates viewed
their educational experience and how they thought it influenced their
own clinical practice after graduation.

Design

The design for the study was qualitative description influenced by
grounded theory. As characterized by Sandelowski (2000), qualitative
description is an established method that allows the researcher to produce a basic description without requiring him or her to provide an
abstract or conceptual explanation of the data. Though all descriptive
studies involve interpretation, qualitative description does not require
the degree of abstract interpretation found in, for example, phenomenology. In other words, the description is produced in everyday terms.

A useful way of looking at the distinction between qualitative description and other approaches is to briefly compare it to another
method, such as narrative analysis. Imagine a set of interviews made up
of stories. The researcher engaged in qualitative description analyzes
the stories in terms of their content—what do the participants say the
story is about, and what are the commonalities and differences in the
content among stories? The researcher may also be interested in describing what happened during the gathering of the interviews, producing field notes on this context that subsequently become part of the
data. The aim is to describe what is contained within the stories.

Narrative analysis, on the other hand, has a different aim. It "examines the informant's story and analyzes how it is put together, the linguis-
tic and cultural resources it draws on, and how it persuades a listener
of authenticity. Analysis in narrative studies opens up the form of telling
about experience, not simply the content to which language refers. We
ask, why was the story told *that* way?" (Riessmann, 1993).

One of the ways our qualitative descriptive study takes on grounded theory overtones arises from our concern with interaction and with the meaning people make of their experiences through social interaction. Grounded theory is based in symbolic interactionism, and several of the key ideas of this conceptual framework have informed our work. We hold certain assumptions about learning, among them that learning is a process that takes place through social interaction. Interactions between and among learners, teachers, patients, preceptors, and places of practice create the spaces and times where learning occurs. As Bowers (1988) explains, the symbolic interactionist believes that we construct our social worlds, and that our roles are built from our interactions with that social world.

MacDonald & Schreiber (2001) state it this way: "Human interaction/action, and the constitution and reconstruction of meaning within levels of context, are central phenomena of interest . . . This is a synergistic and dynamic process in which action/interaction changes the context, which leads, in turn, to the construction of new meanings and new actions" (p. 42).

Though these are all-important ideas for us, and have influenced the way we teach, we did not create a grounded theory study. At this stage of our research, we wanted to describe the experience from the graduates' perspective and begin to see what, if any, influence on practice the graduates would ascribe to the way they learned in class. We present the background on symbolic interactionism because it is part of our cognitive frame, and we wanted to acknowledge and account for this frame in our analysis. Thus, we proposed a qualitative descriptive study to investigate the following questions: (a) How do graduates describe their experiences in the Narrative-Centered Curriculum? (b) How do these learning experiences influence subsequent clinical practice?

Participants

The circumstance of having graduated from our FNP program predetermined the group from which we could draw participants. The group in this instance is small, numbering 73 graduates in the first four years of the program. Our sampling plan was purposive and simple. Our research questions were aimed at all graduates, and we were not attempting to compare or contrast these graduates with any other group. This plan was reasonable, in light of the design and questions.

Thirty-two graduates of the family nurse practitioner program at our school agreed to participate in our study, representing 44% of the available group. Thirty were women, and two were men. Thirty-one were Caucasian, and one woman was of Native American descent. The gender and ethnicity composition of the sample were representative of the larger population of FNP graduates from our school. All were interviewed one year after graduation, and all were working as nurse practitioners. We mailed consent forms to those who expressed interest in being in the study, and the receipt of a signed consent prompted the data gatherers to make an appointment for an interview.

Data Gathering

We chose a relatively unstructured interview format for data gathering. Since our research aim was to describe graduates' experiences of being in the program, we needed extensive information. Yet we didn't want to limit their recollections to any specific part of the program, and since we weren't looking for particular variables, a structured or semistructured interview would not have been helpful.

The data gatherers were research assistants who were also students in the master's program but who were unacquainted with the FNP graduates. We worked extensively with each research assistant, teaching them about conducting interviews, asking opening questions, using conversational probes, and avoiding leading questions. Each of the two assistants was responsible for gathering data from two groups of graduates. We used research assistants to gather data because even though we had close contact with all of the graduates during and after their completion of the program, we felt they would be more comfortable sharing their experiences with interviewers than with faculty.

We also chose to conduct the interviews via the telephone. The main limitation of this approach was that the data gatherers could not see nonverbal responses, and thus we were unable to access visual data that might have been valuable. On the other hand, our graduates are located all over the state, and telephone interviews made it possible to talk with those at a distance. Since we had limited financial support for the study, we had no funds to pay for travel. The decision to use phone interviews seemed the best possible solution given our circumstances.

At the beginning of the first interview the consent was reviewed, and participants had the opportunity to ask questions and to withdraw from the study if they chose. Interviewers invited participants to tell stories about their educational experiences and the effect those experiences had on their subsequent practice as family nurse practitioners. Interviews were recorded on audiotape and transcribed verbatim. Interviewers listened to the tapes while reviewing the transcripts and corrected any errors in the transcriptions. Any notes made by the interviewers were also transcribed and considered as data. Participants were assigned a code number, and the key with names and codes was kept in a locked file cabinet in the office of one of the investigators. Following correction of the transcriptions, tapes were also kept in a locked file cabinet. Upon completion of the study, the tapes were erased. Though participants did vary in their ability to be narratively active, none had difficulty thinking of stories about their experiences in the program.

Data Analysis

Another way in which grounded theory influenced this study was in our data analysis methods. We used the methods of constant comparative analysis outlined by Glaser & Strauss (1967), Glaser (1992), and by Lincoln & Guba (1985). We chose constant comparison because it is an excellent way to organize and work through data analysis (it enabled us to collapse initial analytic ideas into larger themes) while staying close to the text (a requirement for descriptive validity).

We began with open coding, where meaning units of text were labeled with codes taken from the participant's own words. An example of this is the code "knowing where to look." It is important to note that we did not code line by line; rather we looked specifically for meaning units within stories of experiences as both a student and a clinician. We counted both a simple "telling what happened" and more carefully thought-out, more metaphoric and reflective narratives as stories. We moved back and forth through each interview, searching for additional meaning units and for instances of codes that had already been used. We began to develop themes that went beyond the level of the codes, which we tracked with analytic memos. We use "analytic memo," however, slightly differently from the way the term is typically used in grounded theory. Since we were not looking for a theoretical explanation in the data, our memos were not explorations of theoretical notions, but rather ideas for integrating the content descriptions into a higher level of description. Obviously, such memos serve the same purpose as theoretical memos, but more accurately reflect the qualitative descriptive design.

As we moved through our constant comparison, we worked toward a higher level of analysis, attempting to identify the salient features of each story and to establish the relationships between and among story features. Our analytic memos documented our changing ideas and helped us to fill in gaps in data collection and analysis. We also acknowledged our own understandings in the analysis. We explicated our ideas about teaching and learning, our values as teachers, nurses, and nurse practitioners, and discussed our educational and philosophic leanings toward pragmatism and phenomenology. We began to connect our emerging themes to other literature on narratives, listening, and interpretation. The discussion that follows details the central theme developed through our analysis: *Listening to Learn*. Constant comparison became a way to build and structure our description rather than a way to discover a basic social process or core variable, as would be true in grounded theory.

Establishing Quality

Since the assumptions of qualitative research differ so greatly from the assumptions of traditional scientific research, the quality criteria also must differ. This study used guidelines developed by the researchers and modified from many authors' ideas (Lincoln, 1995; Lincoln & Denzin, 1994; 1997; Noddings, 1984; Patton, 1999; Sandelowski, 2000; Schwandt, 1996). Our suggestions abandon the conventional scientific criteria of objectivity, reliability, validity, and generalizability, and go beyond the analogous criteria proposed by Lincoln & Guba (1989, p. 236–243): credibility, dependability, transferability, and confirmability. Table 3.2 summarizes our ideas about quality criteria.

Sandelowski (2000) outlines two essential elements of qualitative description: descriptive validity and interpretive validity. Descriptive validity refers to the accuracy of the accounts, and interpretive validity refers to an "accurate accounting of the meanings participants attributed to those events" (p. 336). We addressed descriptive validity by cross-checking transcripts with tapes. In addition, the techniques of constant comparison are specifically designed to keep the researcher close to the data when generating descriptions of events. Interpretive validity goes further than descriptive validity. Both researchers and one research assistant coded all transcripts and met frequently to discuss and resolve differences in description and interpretation. We also held several

Table 3.2 Proposed Quality Criteria

Criterion	How we seek to achieve the criterion
Consistency	We seek consistency between and among the research paradigm, the research questions, the research methods, and the research conclusions. Each of these drives subsequent research activities. In a qualitative descriptive study, the questions are of the "who, what, why, when" variety, the data gathering and analysis techniques attempt to produce the fullest possible description without resulting in methodologically driven interpretations, and the conclusions are presented in descriptive, rather than theoretical, terms.
Coherence	The study "holds together," flows logically and cogently, and makes sense. Other clinical teachers find the study resonates with their own experiences.
Clarity	The research report defines any ambiguous terms, seeks plainness and simplicity of construction, and tries to explain findings using terminology germane to the discipline.
Conscious Connected-ness:	We seek to stay connected with the participants in the study, including students, teachers, and clinicians. We also seek to make meaningful connections to the literature in nursing, clinical education, philosophy, and pedagogy.
Credibility	By describing our situation fully, by documenting our conclusions using clear text examples, and by our prolonged engagement with the respondents and the texts, we hope to present a study that is believable, with conclusions that can be depended upon for their accuracy. We present ourselves as qualified researchers, with experience in a variety of qualitative and interpretive methods.
Collaboration	We seek to present the authentic voices of our graduates, and extend to them our gratitude for their willingness to participate in this study. They are co-creators of the findings.
Fairness	All voices are represented, including contrasting viewpoints.
Usefulness	By this we mean applicability, transferability, practical benefit to teachers, learners, clinical preceptors, practitioners, and ultimately, patients and families. Descriptions of approaches and strategies, examples of written work and assignments, an outline of a traditional curriculum contrasted with the Narrative-Centered Curriculum, and presentation of our own reflections on the study are intended to make possible the adaptation of our ideas by other teachers in other situations.

informal discussions with graduates, who thought our interpretations were accurate.

We propose that this study demonstrates consistency and coherence between questions and methods to preserve the epistemological integrity of the project. This includes consistency of research paradigm, research questions, methods of data collection and analysis, as well as results and evaluation of results. We strive for clarity through unambiguous statements of assumptions and purpose, explicit descriptions of methods of data collection and analysis, and avoidance of jargon. We propose that this study demonstrates a conscious connectedness between the voices of the participants and the interpretations of the researchers. We present data and descriptions that are believable, conclusions that resonate with the reality of the reader, and an effective interpretation of the findings within the context. We have endeavored to demonstrate fairness by presenting conclusions constructed from the voices of the participants, giving weight to no particular view. Finally, we present this study with an emphasis on its usefulness to teachers, clinicians, and clinical students, keeping in mind that new pedagogies are always site-specific and always mediated by context. Our own personal research values include empathy (for research participants), collaboration (with participants and with colleagues and critics), and a commitment to the potential usefulness of the study for participants and readers, since we desire to present new knowledge based on experience about practices that are helpful.

Discussion of Findings

We entered into the study knowing that we were interested in Narrative Pedagogy, experience-based learning, and the connections between the two. We also wanted to look at how learning influenced the practices of clinicians after graduation. Working with the transcript data, we constructed two areas of focus: learning in a new way and listening in a new way. We connected these ideas to develop the theme *Listening to Learn*.

Learning in a New Way

Students struggled with learning to think in a new way from the very first course in the major, even though they had been accustomed to

extensive use of structured case study analysis in both their pathophysiology and pharmacology courses. In the physical assessment course,
however, they were presented with patients who narrated a history regarding a specified issue or health problem, rather than a case study.
Faculty first modeled the listening role by obtaining the history; later,
student volunteers elicited the patient's history. This approach prepared
them for their later courses, which used modified Practice-Based Learning approaches and other narrative experiences as the basis for every
class session. After pathophysiology, pharmacology, and physical assessment, teachers never lectured. Melody, who graduated two years ago,
described her experiences in the narrative classroom this way:

> In class, it wasn't lecture and then a test. It was more real problems and thinking
> through, and thought-processing and learning in a different way. And I enjoyed
> that, I appreciated that. I know some people who were wondering if we were
> learning as much as we should, but there is so much to learn that I don't think
> any method can give you everything that there is you need to know. We had
> to be responsible for getting that on our own. I enjoyed the method of learning,
> and it serves me very well, every time I walk into a room to see a patient. I
> learned to listen and to care.

Melody responded positively to learning with stories and found that stories helped her in her clinical practice after leaving the program. She
understood that narratives are reconstructions of lived experience and
that her ability to listen to patients enhanced her nursing practice. She
felt that she had been guided to learn what she needed to learn, rather
than being given what she needed to know.

However, a very few of her classmates were not as entirely satisfied.
They were concerned because the culture of the classroom didn't "give
them everything there is that you need to know." The craving for structure reveals their familiarity with traditional pedagogies. An example
from Adrian follows:

> [The program] has a very unstructured way of teaching, and I understand that
> they are trying to evolve a new method of teaching with the practice-based
> approach and learning from stories, but I still think that you have to give us,
> we still have to have a little structure to it. I think they need to have a case
> on, like, there is only one way to treat urinary tract infections: you do this, this,
> and this. And it is not to teach cookbook method of practice, but to teach a
> whole process of learning that [the faculty] is trying to do. I have to have a
> protocol. In fact, that is one of the things that won the physician over that is

my medical director. He wanted to know if I had a book of protocols on what nurse practitioners did, and I actually had just been to the bookstore and had found a book. It's a book of protocols for ambulatory care or something. It's step one, two, three, four, and five of what a nurse practitioner would go through and it gives at the bottom when to refer to a physician. That's all it took for me to win him over to show him that I was not trying to replace him, but it was still a, b, c, d, e. We were both more comfortable with more structure and clear direction. My particular class was too free form, and I am an easy, adaptable person. Not much makes me nervous, but there were times when I felt like I was struggling trying to stay afloat in school because there was no structure to it.

Although most students seemed to be able to disconnect from old habits of learning, some never could. Their ways of thinking were little changed, and even though they assimilated critical content and are now competent practitioners, they demonstrated a low tolerance for the ambiguity of clinical practice. Fortunately, they were able to find places of employment that provided them with the structure they wished for and needed. Even when students beg for instructional scaffolding, they acknowledge that structure cannot provide all the answers. The published medical protocols Adrian cherishes do offer answers to clearly identified medical situations, but fail to provide individualized, personal solutions for specific patients and families. Nevertheless, Adrian finds comfort in the protocol book.

Gloria, one of our first year graduates, on the other hand, shows that students can recognize new ways of learning. She especially mentions that narratives provided her with knowledge she could remember and apply in practice:

I did learn a different way of thinking about patient care. I was prepared to take the [national certification] exam. I was successful in passing the exam, and as I have gotten started in doing some practice here and there, I find a lot of what I learned coming back to me. The way we learned, that was different because it was all around stories from patients and other students, that way sticks with you and you remember things. I will always remember those patients' stories.

Because the learning is connected to the experience of the individual patient story, it becomes part of the vicarious experience of the learner. It is memorable and therefore, useful.

Jeff, a community health nurse who had years of experience before he entered graduate school, found that learning from the classroom stories of patients motivated him to go beyond what was required in his reading and thinking:

I felt that learning by patient's stories, I probably studied harder than had I been told to sit down and read a bunch of chapters. You know, instead of having to read an assignment, I probably went off on more side trails looking up interesting and useful things that I could apply in practice, information I wanted and needed to know more than just looking up straight facts. My patients don't read books, none of them follow the textbooks, and I think no lecture can prepare you for real patients who don't read the textbooks and their bodies don't read the textbooks and no patient has just one thing going on with them. That is why I think the case stories were really useful because you got a broader picture of what was going on with a real person than if you had just studied heart disease or kidney disease, or if you had just read the chapter and thought of it as an isolated body system. I felt it was a more integrated, a more real-life learning experience than the traditional read-the-chapters-and-take-the-test type of learning.

Jeff articulated how the classroom experience was transformed in the clinical arena. He pointed out that he was able to connect his own interpretation of patients' stories with his skilled nursing practices after graduation, noting especially that he carefully and reflectively attended to all the concerns of his patients. Jeff was able to take the learning he generated for himself and use it in practice to recognize the not-so-classic patient presentation, the unique situation. He was able to separate the patient from the disease and to see each person as an individual with a story to relate about health and illness.

Listening in a New Way

Tabitha related her skills as a listener and showed how her classroom experiences with listening to the whole story were helpful to her and to her patient:

Well, I'll give you a story example of how the curriculum helps me every day. It had to do with an older woman, a 72-year-old woman, who had come in several times, seen both the physicians that I work with in the practice, and then scheduled with me. When I walked into the room, I had never met this woman before in my life, the woman wouldn't talk to me at first. She was just seething with anger, and so it took me awhile to get her to warm up and to tell me what was going on. I had to give her time. I had to show her she could trust me to listen to her and not try to tell her right away what was wrong with her. Anyway, this woman had progressively over a 6-week period gone from a very independent, very active life to having almost constant pain. She was even having difficulty walking. She was having hip pain and joint pain. They just told her that she had arthritis and gave her anti-inflammatory drugs. I listened to this women for a long time and ended up diagnosing her with polymyalgia, which they had missed. I put her on steroids and she was a new woman, so of course she thought I was wonderful, but it was an example of actually taking the time to listen to this woman and to hear the whole story. As a fairly new practitioner, I picked up something because I listened to her so carefully. Maybe it was because I had more time to spend with this woman, more time to pay attention.

Tabitha shows that one of her skilled practices involves taking the time to listen to the patient. The listening she describes is engaged and active, aimed at more than just "getting the history." Adler (1997) would characterize this kind of listening as a way of being a therapeutic presence for the patient as well as a means to a more accurate diagnosis.

Lucy remembered vividly how stories were communicated among student, teachers, and patients. She refers to both oral and written stories in this comment:

Well, it was good in that you could learn a lot from each other, because we all came from different backgrounds, there was time to share that within the class. There was always communication, oh, how do I want to say . . . communication was always encouraged to voice our opinion and when opinions were voiced by people who had different experiences, that helped us all. Everybody listened to everybody, and learned from them. The stories really put it all there for me. Of all the things that I perceived about the program, reading those stories is one of the things that I found to be the most exciting.

This nurse practitioner makes clear that narratives shared in class enabled a collaborative learning experience. The stories "put it all there" for her and for her classmates and teachers. Stories served a unifying function that helped her learn from the experiences of others, accessed by listening. Presumably, there is communication in all classrooms, even in asynchronous internet-based virtual classrooms. Why, then, does this graduate (and many others) choose to remember the level, kind, and meaning of storied communication in her educational experience? Perhaps it is not simple communication she remembers, but rather the dialogue present in the classroom that is more than speaking and hearing, the meaningful dialogue that provides a basis for authentic relationships enabling learning.

Listening and hearing the meanings inherent in words is a skill that most advanced practice nursing curricula do not address in any systematic way. Faculty members may assume that students acquired listening skills in the course of their baccalaureate education and that they have retained and polished these skills over the years. Unfortunately, we have found that graduate students in nursing have lost their listening abilities, indeed may have deliberately abandoned these skills in favor of more fundamentally pragmatic technical skills and multi-tasking. We find students to be rather self-absorbed at the beginning the program, striving to be detached and objective in their dealings with patients. Anything not absolutely connected to the problem on which they are focused is dismissed as irrelevant.

However, later in the program, and after graduation, they are able to demonstrate an attentive willingness to listen. This listening requires an openness to the other that is critical to human understanding and response. Gadamer writes (1982, p. 324):

In human relations, the important thing is . . . to experience the [other] and not to overlook his claim and listen to what he has to say to us. To this end, openness is necessary. But this openness exists ultimately not only for the person to whom one listens, but rather anyone who listens is fundamentally open. Without this kind of openness to one another there is no genuine human relationship. Belonging together always also means being able to listen to one another.

Fiumara (1990) suggests that "listening is the attitude which can unblock the creative resources immobilized by the rigidity of traditional, 'logical' education" (p. 165). But to develop a listening attitude requires a willingness to change the way we are, to transform ourselves through learning. It is much more than memorizing lists of differential diagnoses, appropriate drug management, and laboratory tests. Listening opens the student, the teacher, and the clinician to possibilities of experience that are not attainable any other way, always remembering those patients' stories.

Listening fully and reflectively is a skill and art that must be demonstrated, practiced, discussed, and refined. Listening that is intent, active, involved, and open to the other has not been emphasized in nurse practitioner education; we find this a dangerous omission. Centering our pedagogies on narratives, which are written, spoken, read, and listened to, shows our commitment to listening as a valuable aspect of advanced practice nursing. Without interpretive listening, remembering may be imperfect. Clinical practice may be competent, but the clinician who lacks listening ability may depend more heavily on the scaffolding of pre-determined protocols.

When students are open to hearing the full narrative of a patient's concern, they are less likely to jump to diagnostic conclusions, less likely to overlook issues that are priorities for the patient, and less likely to assume that they know what is "going on" even before the patient has explained the situation. Heidegger (1990) suggests in *On the Way to Language* that it "might be helpful to us to rid ourselves of the habit of only hearing what we already understand" (p. 58). Eleana related this story about a breakdown in listening and how she learned from her mistake:

I did have quite an interesting experience when [my clinical instructor] made her last visit of the summer when I was completing my residency. She was waiting on me to complete a situation that I was in with a patient. It was a well-child check and the mom had brought the little girl in. It was a Monday morning and this was a teenage mom. I don't know if she was even 18 yet. She worked nights. She had just come off the night shift and picked up her little girl. She had been gone all weekend with her boyfriend and came home, went to work, got home and found her little girl sick. And so I was dealing with a sick child, and when I got to the ear exam, of course, the baby cried and cried and the next thing I knew the mom was shoving everything into her diaper bag and she says, "I'm leaving. You made my baby cry. The doctor never makes my baby cry. I'm leaving." And out the door she went, stomping and slamming the door. And I asked her to come back. I said, "Well, wait, I'll go get my preceptor. I'll go get the doctor. Your baby's got an ear infection and needs to be treated." "No, I'm leaving." And she stomped out the door. You know, and I thought what did I do wrong? I felt terrible. And [my instructor] was very supportive and said, "Well, you know, these things happen to everyone, and not just to students." And the physician was very nice and very supportive and called the mom and apparently, well, I think she felt guilty for having been gone all weekend and the child was ill when she got back and she was very tired. She hadn't been to bed yet, and that in combination with she apparently had no recollection of the baby crying when someone examined her ears before, plus the baby had an ear infection and she was worried. So that was very, you know, unsettling to me and to her. Very upsetting, actually, because I didn't really listen to what she was concerned about. I learned a lot from that. Well, in fact, what I do now before I look at any kid's ear, I find out the whole story of how much the child has been upsetting the family routine and all. Whether the mom has gotten any sleep with the sick baby. I give her a chance to talk about it and I <u>let her know that I am listening to her.</u>

Eleana provides an example of what happens when there is a lapse in listening. She heard only what she expected to hear, ignoring the unsaid and missing an opportunity to connect with a tired mother. She shows how students become unmindful of some skills as they focus on others, and how distraction and anxiety can interfere with their ability to listen to the patient. Despite all the talk about listening that occurs in the classroom, when it came to demonstrating skilled listening comportment in the clinical setting, the student focused on the doing instead. Nevertheless, she was able to learn from this breakdown in communication and use it to change her practice in the future.

The listening that students engaged in required their cognitive, emotional, and intentional presence. It also required them to develop the ability to notice and understand nuances in language, actions, silence, rhythm, and theme, as well as the ability to listen beyond the language to the meaning evoked. It is an artful listening, in every sense of the word. It is listening on purpose and listening with purpose.

Taking the time to listen, and then to reflectively consider the meaning of the words, helps students to be a therapeutic presence at the same time they collect data for a differential diagnosis. We encourage students to become "apprentices of listening, rather than masters of discourse" (Fiumara, 1990, p. 57). Listening must be learned, and students must be shown how to listen in a new way so that they hear beyond the words to the meaning. "A listening atmosphere is not improvised. It is, on the contrary, the product of a strenuous process of conception, growth, and devoted attention" (Fiumara, 1990, p. 60). In the Narrative-Centered Curriculum, where we emphasize hearing the meaning of words, listening with presence is critically important because listening is the "other side of language" (Fiumara, 1990). Without listening to the language, words mean little. Listening requires the clinician stop talking, to create sufficient open silence to allow himself or herself to hear what the patient needs to tell. A listening attitude, a listening silence, allows us to listen (in spite of the din of the dominant culture [Fiumara, 1990, p. 95]).

Philip came to the program with an extensive emergency room nursing background. In his career, he had repeatedly been rewarded for being a "fast diagnoser." He prided himself on being able to know what the problem was even before the patient related a single symptom. He struggled to learn to take time with patients, to hear what concerned them, before making his diagnostic decisions. After graduation, he looked back on his experiences this way:

I think the narrative way is a good way to learn. I liked it. Lectures get boring and then it is difficult to remember what is covered. I did more research and more studying than with traditional lecture courses. I am a "clinical" thinker, so I learned more from the clinical stories in class. Our paradigm story write-ups took a long time, but I learned a lot from having to put all that thinking down on paper, especially the part about writing in your own words, which was pretty hard to do. The stories we listened to and discussed improved my analytical thinking and my thinking in depth about what patients were really concerned about.

In a world of ever more information and concern with detail, it would be easy to rationalize the need to continually expand knowledge at the expense of deeply knowing our selves, our students, and our patients. Listening makes clear what is important, which details can be set aside, and where attention should be focused. In the long run, this approach can save time in a busy practice day, rather than take up too much of it. It can save us from seeing only that which we already understand and can prevent us from succumbing to the myth that our patients are mirror images of ourselves.

A critical element of narrative pedagogies is teachers modeling learning to listen with students and with one another. Stories unheard are as nonproductive as stories uninterpreted. Deborah adds:

I'm an old nurse and so I knew what my philosophy was, so I knew I would have that same philosophy as an advanced practice nurse. And I was heard when I talked about my philosophy, other students listened to me and the faculty listened to me, and that helped me learn to listen to them, too. Listening now to my patients, and really taking the time to listen to them, is probably the most important thing I learned in this program . . . Just being thorough isn't enough, you must be really looking and listening to your patients, that is just so important, and I try never to miss doing that. Patients say, "You listen, you take the time, you seem to really care about me." I don't look at my watch, I don't look at the clock. I don't say "your 15 minutes are up and you've gotta go." They leave with the feeling that, yes, they are important, yes, someone listened to them. The patients love this kind of paying attention to their concerns. Listening IS the medicine for many of my patients.

Moustakas (1995) writes of the listening that occurs during a therapy session: "To really know another person in significant moments of that person's life, I listen to the range of voices, the variations of speech, the tones and textures, sounds of joy and anger, the mixture of sadness and laughter, the edgy, uncertain words of fear, the myriad facial and body expressions . . . the lengthy silences and continuous stream of words . . . and all the ups and downs of ecstasy and misery" (p. 57). Moustakas refers to listening of a particular type—the psychotherapist listening to a patient. Though the content of psychological narratives may be different from narratives heard in a family practice (sometimes), the listening practice is the same. It is the complete attentiveness to what shows itself in the conversation, paying attention to the liminal spaces between what is said and what is not said, to discover what is meant.

Listening to Learn

Stories that enable one to engage vicariously in the experiences of others are the connections between people and experiences that enable learning. This is the heart of the central theme, *Listening to Learn*. Selina illustrates how she makes this connection when she comments on the experiential aspects of the narrative curriculum. She was able to internalize the experiences of the stories shared in the classroom and in her writing and reading. For Selina, the activities of listening created the link between experiencing the narrative and making it part of her own practice life.

I just think the way that we did case studies and stories and listened to stories and talked more about real life experiences than just doing like didactic type course work . . . was a much better way to learn. It seems more like real life, more like what really happens in clinical practice. . . . I think that you just forget so much if all you're doing is sitting in a lecture-type format all the time. I think I just learned a lot better by having the information related to real human experience versus just stuff written on a board or something that you copied notes from. Stories from the actual patients are better ways to learn how to listen and think about what the person is saying about what is important to them. . . . We learned that ability to see and listen to a person as a whole. The ability to look beyond what might be on the surface, and that skill came from stories, I think. Our research projects helped this too, because they were qualitative research and we had to learn how to listen during an interview and how to not jump to conclusions. Listening to and absorbing the life stories, they become a part of my experience and me. Seeing the patient and family at their most vulnerable and weakest times, and sometimes at their best, draws me into their world with an intensity that often only nurses have been privileged to feel. Listening to their life experiences links me to them. The power of their words describes their roller coaster experiences and the overwhelming constraints in their lives. I will take their words with me as I move in and out of other patients' lives. I will listen more carefully to hear exactly what their illness means to them and their families.

Our students construct themselves as listeners and interpreters of stories. As they do, they also construct their own autobiographies as practitioners. If Bruner (1990) is correct, these listening and interpretive practices become the means by which they structure their clinical experiences and project themselves into the future as listening practitioners.

Ursula K. Le Guin, a novelist and short story writer, wrote about how stories are transferred from teller to hearer: "By remembering it, he makes the story his. Insofar as I have remembered it, it is mine; and now, if you like it, it's yours. In the tale, in the telling, we are all one blood" (1981, p. 195). By remembering the story and interpreting it, and later by telling it, the student is able to make it a permanent part of her or his experience, thereby rendering it available and useful. The story inextricably connects the teller and the listener. To remember the story is not just to apply knowledge and skills to practice. It is more than pattern matching, adherence to clinical guidelines, or just knowing what, and is even more than knowing how. Advanced practice nursing, carried out using attentive listening, is an interpretive practice. Professional reflection is characteristic of skilled comportment and caring practice.

Self-reflection involves listening to one's own story of what one wants to become and how one wants to shape one's practice. This inner listening (Fiumara, 1990, p. 127) is the capacity for listening to one's self, hearing the ways one knows and understands, and explaining one's responses and interpretations. Stories allow students to engage vicariously in experiences of others and to learn from their own narratives as they reflect on the meaning of the words and the ways in which particular words transform thinking. According to Frank (1995):

Thinking with stories means joining with them. . . . The goal is empathy, not as internalizing the feelings of the other, but resonance with the other. The other's self story does not become my own, but I develop sufficient resonance with that story so that I can feel its nuances and anticipate changes. . . . When stories are retold, the point is not only what is learned from their content. . . . The point is rather what a listener *becomes* in the course of listening to the story. Repetition is the medium of becoming. Professional culture has little space for personal becoming. The problem is truly to *listen* to one's own story, just as the problem is truly to listen to other's stories. (pp. 158–159)

Frank's message to health professionals is that the clinician is not at the center of the universe. Patients don't tell us things for our benefit or our learning; rather, they tell us for their own benefit. Even so, the listener is always changed by truly listening to another's story; the very interaction between the listener and the teller becomes part of the listener's autobiography and lays the ground for how she will listen in the future. In the literal sense, the patient's story becomes part of the nurse practitioner's story of herself or himself as a helping professional. If a patient tells the story of his headaches, and if the clinician really listens to him, together they can construct a way to make sense of the experience and solve the problem; it becomes part of the clinician's identity and informs how she practices, as well as part of the patient's ongoing story of experiences in the healthcare system. It can even play a part in what way the patient decides to seek help (or not) in the future. Telling that story to a student or another clinician enables them to learn from it and make it their own as well. All share the common meaning of the story, but also make unique sense of it as individuals. These stories echo through the experiences of numerous people, changing each one who truly hears it, and becoming changed in the process.

Likewise, dialogue in education depends entirely on the relationship between the participants. Teachers who listen can be transformed by their students' stories. The authentic dialogue that occurs between an alert listener and an engaged storyteller informs how both will listen in the future. Teachers must demonstrate an openness to listening that invites a trusting dialogue with students. It follows, then, that by demonstrating an openness to listening with patients and clinical preceptors students can establish and preserve a caring relationship. We can respond to the other with our presence, with our true listening, or we can be there but not present. In the same way, students can sit passively in class, appearing to listen to lecture or seminar conversation. But because they are disengaged, or because they want to hear what they already understand, or they want to be told exactly what to do, they are unable to attach any meaning to the narrative. In a situation demanding mindful listening, they find themselves dissatisfied, perhaps because their preferred passive mode of learning has been challenged.

Summary and Implications

The central theme, *Listening to Learn*, resonates with Epstein's (1999) ideas regarding mindful practice in medicine. He included active observation of oneself, the patient, and the presenting issue; a willingness to examine and set aside prejudices and predetermined categories; attention to the connection between the knower and the known; compassion built on insight; a commitment to providing a listening presence; reflection and critical self-evaluation; and an openness to the possibilities inherent in the patient-clinician relationship. We have focused on aspects of storytelling, story listening, and story interpretation as a means of teaching nurse practitioner students how to be aware of their way of being in their work as clinicians.

How can these approaches be used in other disciplines and at other levels of learning? Narrative pedagogies are site-specific; each teacher must evaluate each learning situation to make self-reflective decisions about pedagogical choices. We are indeed fortunate to have graduate students in small classes. These are highly motivated, self-directed learners who are already professionals and who have a thirst for learning.

We know teachers who have used Problem-Based Learning, Practice-Based Learning (Barrows, 1994), and other forms of experience-based learning in large groups of novices. In these cases, smaller groups form and re-form within the classroom community, with instructors/tutors circulating between and among the groups. When large groups are presented with issues, more structure often helps define the boundaries of the problem, and the discussion can focus on one aspect at time. Novices often need help in distinguishing what is important from what is merely anecdotally interesting; making this distinction is the job of the teacher, who provides an organizing template for problem-solving.

Large class sections are efficient, but their use is often determined by economic considerations rather than by a desire to employ an effective pedagogy. Breaking a large group into more intimate sections, even for a few minutes during a class session, may make the difference between an instructional factory approach to education and an approach grounded in listening and learning.

We have given up the prepared lecture because it fails to provide a way for students to generate their own knowledge. When we lecture, we fail to listen. Students also fail to listen as they sit passively in the classroom, frantically taking notes on our every word but not hearing what we say. Of course the lecture is not, in itself, damaging. We all have attended lectures we thought were informative, stimulating, challenging, and entertaining. The lecture is an art form when done well. What is dangerous is the complacent failure to reflect on teaching and the failure to consider innovative approaches to teaching and learning. Always to prefer to lecture may indicate that the teacher has not taken time to reflect on teaching. Depending entirely on the familiar format of the lecture may encourage teachers to fail to consider other, more innovative, approaches to teaching and learning. Lecturing, to the exclusion of other, more interactive methods, may discourage students from developing their own ways of generating knowledge and may slow their progress toward critical thinking and their own professional reflection.

Lectures are not the problem, but rather how teachers lecture. What worries us is that when one lectures, one is not listening to others (Young & Diekelmann, 2002). The lecture, by its very definition, promotes teacher-centered instruction. The dominant culture in higher education, which manifests itself in traditional, teacher-centered pedagogies, is the culture of non-present non-listening. We propose dialogical classrooms and clinical settings in which teachers listen as much as students do and in which both can listen to learn. We encourage students to listen also to the pages of their texts, by which we mean they ought to be mindful readers, always preserving the contexts that circle the stories of illness and health. This classroom ought to be neither teacher-centered nor student-centered, but centered on listening practices that promote thinking and making meaning.

If stories told by students, teachers, patients, and clinicians call forth listening, and if listening calls forth meaning, why are we not listening more closely to one another? Which practices of telling, listening, and interpreting can co-occur in classrooms and clinical experiences? How can we recognize, demonstrate, and teach listening practices? Could we teach, and could our students learn, a culture of listening? Fiumara (1990) suggests, "There is no such thing as a method of learning to listen to something" (p. 49). And yet, our students do learn to listen and do listen to learn. Stories keep this possibility open and alive in our classroom. This is where the usefulness of the study shows itself: it reveals that narrative pedagogies are the link between listening and learning.

This is a very slow revolution for us and for our colleagues in nursing. We explore alternative ways of thinking, finding meaning, and interpreting knowledge in our classroom, but we do not entirely denigrate the teaching done in other classrooms using a more conventional pedagogy. These traditional (and usually behaviorist) environments require that the teacher select and sequence the content, plan all the learning events, and decide whether the desired learning has taken place. Lectures are content driven, tests are formal and objective, and grading is rigid. We propose a shift to a pedagogy of meaning-in-context, where students critique, explore, and deconstruct their own experiences and those of others to magnify the relevance and grounded nature of their learning. What is important is that we continue the conversation with our colleagues to promote mutual critique and reflection on teaching and learning. We must be open to all new possibilities, or we will continue to teach as we were taught, which may be harmful to ourselves and our students.

What paradigm a teacher chooses to use is determined by the goals of the teaching, of the school, and of the students. Our goal is informed and competent practice, but beyond that, we seek understanding, which is knowledge in a meaningful context. Without meaning-in-context, information is stagnant and virtually useless in the long run. We use aspects of the instructional paradigm, such as testing, but we reconfigure and reform tests to promote new learning rather than simply to evaluate knowledge of content. We use multiple-choice tests, but we present these as take-home tests, to be researched for the rationale behind each answer choice. We ask questions related to issues not previously discussed in class.

We want to make it possible for graduate clinical-education students to transfer their classroom thinking directly to practice, easily and quickly. Using narrative and experience-based approaches, we have de-

emphasized teacher control of content and focused on creating meaningful learning and reflective clinical practice through listening and dialogue. We have evaluated every course at its conclusion, evaluated every
cohort at graduation, interviewed graduates and preceptors, and talked
with employers. Students completing the major have been successful in
achieving national certification (92% on first try, 100% on second try,
compared to a national average of approximately 80%) and in gaining
employment as advanced practice nurses.

The results of our aim to decenter content and emphasize the power
of stories are apparent in our students years after they graduate. They
are able to see that their learning experiences have transformed the
ways they think about patient care and about their own practice. They
are able to articulate personal goals of listening and learning, which they
continue to strive to achieve. Graduates have internalized the values of
the program when they recognize that every patient, every family, and
every clinician has a story worth hearing, worth reflecting on, and worth
incorporating into clinical practice.

Conclusion

Although we regard our approaches to teaching and learning as a
work in progress, we are confident about the value of narrative and reflective approaches in nurse practitioner clinical education (Young &
Diekelmann, 2002; Diekelmann, 2000; Diekelmann, 2001). We believe
these strategies will reduce unthinking adherence to a purely rational-
technical model of care and augment it with a new approach of listening-
to-learn reflective nursing practice. Reform begins at the most basic
instructional level, teacher-by-teacher, course-by-course, classroom-by-
classroom. Incremental changes make possible entirely new pedagogies.
The site-specific approaches teachers choose absolutely influence the
quality of clinical practice. Narrative pedagogies, as shown in this study,
allow an educational culture that rests in the authentic openness required to sustain a revealing and meaningful dialogue between teacher
and student, student and preceptor, clinician and patient.

Notes

1. Our definition of narrative goes beyond the structured and unstructured story to
include narrative thinking about personal and vicarious experiences that can be the ob-

jects of reflection in the service of learning. Narratives are the deliberate and mindful reconstruction of experience. Hopkins (1994) refers to a "deep human impulse toward narrative" (p. 10), and this curriculum focuses on narrative as a means of connecting experience with learning.

2. A curriculum, by our definition, is not a "thing" that can be picked up and moved, intact, to another educational situation. The curriculum is not separable from a specific teaching and learning context. Each curriculum is an environmental context, a set of approaches specific to and created by the particular teachers and students involved. Ours could be useful in other settings, but would require modifications if other teachers and learners were to try out it out for themselves.

3. Experiential learning: experience implies "living through." We recognize and celebrate experience as a legitimate learning strategy. Experience can be personal or vicarious, in that the story of the experience remakes it for the teller, and makes it available to the listener. Experience teaches. Narratives connect.

4. Although the teacher has invited the particular person or family to class expecting that a particular story will be told, there is always an element of uncertainty; people tell their own story in their own way, which is not always completely predictable. Charles Sanders Peirce (1976), an American philosopher, wrote: "Experience is our only teacher. And . . . this action of experience . . . takes place by a series of surprises" (p. 37). We are often surprised by whatever experiences the person decides to tell the class, but never sorry that they relate whatever they relate.

References

Adler, H. M. (1997). The history of the present illness as treatment: Who's listening, and why does it matter. *Journal of the American Board of Family Practice, 10*(1), 28–35.

American Association of Colleges of Nursing (1996). *The essentials of master's education for advanced practice nursing.* Washington, DC: American Association of Colleges of Nursing.

Andrews, C. A., Ironside, P. M., Nosek, C., Sims, S. L., Swenson, M. M., Yeomans, C., et al. (2001). Enacting narrative pedagogy: The lived experiences of students and teachers. *Nursing and Health Care Perspectives, 22*(5), 252–259.

Barr, R., & Tagg, J. (1995). From teaching to learning: A new paradigm for undergraduate education. *Change Magazine, 27*(6), 12–25.

Barrows, H. S. (1994). *Practice-based learning: Problem-based learning applied to medical education.* Springfield, IL: Southern Illinois University School of Medicine.

Bateson, M. C. (1994). *Peripheral visions: Learning along the way.* New York: HarperCollins.

Bellack, J. P., Graber, D. R., O'Neil, E. H., Musham, C., & Lancaster, C. (1999). Curriculum trends in nurse practitioner programs: Current and ideal. *Journal of Professional Nursing, 15*(1), 15–27.

Bowers, B. J. (1988). Grounded theory. In B. Sarter (Ed.), *Paths to knowledge: Innovative research methods for nursing.* New York: National League for Nursing Press.

Bruner, J. (1990). *Acts of meaning.* Cambridge, MA: Harvard University Press.

Brykczynski, K. A. (1989). An interpretive study describing the clinical judgment of nurse practitioners. *Scholarly Inquiry for Nursing Practice: An International Journal, 3*(2), 75–104.

Coles, R. (1990). *The call of stories: Teaching and the moral imagination.* New York: Mariner Books.

Dewey, J. (1938). *Experience and education.* New York: Collier Books.

Diekelmann, N. (2000) Being prepared for class: Challenging taken-for-granted assumptions. (Editorial). *Journal of Nursing Education, 39*(7), 291–293.

Diekelmann, N. (2001). Narrative pedagogy: Heideggerian hermeneutical analysis of the lived experience of students, teachers, and clinicians. *Advances in Nursing Science, 23*(3), 53–71.

Diekelmann, N., & Diekelmann, J. (2000). Learning ethics in nursing and genetics: Narrative pedagogy and the grounding of values. *Journal of Pediatric Nursing, 15*(4), 226–231.

Epstein, R. M. (1999). Mindful practice. *Journal of the American Medical Association, 282*(9), 833–839.

Fiumara, G. C. (1990). *The other side of language: A philosophy of listening.* (C. Lambert, Trans.). New York: Routledge.

Frank, A. (1995). *The wounded storyteller: Body, illness, and ethics.* Chicago: University of Chicago Press.

Gadamer, H. G. (1982). *Truth and method.* (G. Barden & J. Cumming, Trans.). New York: Crossroad. (Original German work published in 1960.)

Glaser, B. G. (1992). *Basics of grounded theory analysis: Emergence vs. forcing.* Mill Valley, CA: Sociology Press.

Glaser, B. G., & Strauss, A. L. (1967). *The discovery of grounded theory: Strategies for qualitative research.* Chicago: Aldine.

Heidegger, M. (1971). *On the way to language.* (P. D. Hertz, Trans.). New York: Harper & Row.

Hopkins, R. L. (1994). *Narrative schooling: Experiential learning and the transformation of American education. Advances in Contemporary Educational Thought, 13.* New York: Teachers College Press.

Ironside, P. M. (1999). Thinking in nursing education—Part 1: A student's perspective. *Nursing and Health Care Perspectives, 20*(5), 238–242.

Le Guin, U. K. (1981). "It was a dark and stormy night," or why are we huddling around the campfire? In W. J. T. Mitchell (Ed.), *On narrative.* Chicago: University of Chicago Press.

Lincoln, Y. S. (1995). Emerging criteria for quality in qualitative and interpretive research. *Qualitative Inquiry, 1*(3), 275–289.

Lincoln, Y. S. (1997). What constitutes quality in interpretive research? In C. K. Kinzer, K. A. Hinchman, & D. J. Leu (Eds.), *Inquiries in literacy: Theory and practice.* Chicago: National Reading Conference.

Lincoln, Y. S., & Denzin, N. K. (1994). The fifth moment. In Denzin N. K. and Lincoln, Y. S. (Eds.). *Handbook of qualitative research.* Thousand Oaks, CA: Sage.

Lincoln, Y. S., & Guba, E. G. (1985). *Naturalistic inquiry.* Thousand Oaks, CA: Sage.

Lincoln, Y. S , & Guba, E. G. (2000). Paradigmatic controversies, contradictions, and emerging confluences. In N. K. Denzin & Y. S. Lincoln (Eds.), *Handbook of qualitative research. (2nd Ed.)* Thousand Oaks CA: Sage.

MacDonald, M., & Schreiber, R. S. (2001). Constructing and deconstructing: Grounded theory in a postmodern world. In R. S. Schreiber, & P. N. Stern (Eds.), *Using grounded theory in nursing.* New York: Springer.

Moustakas, C. (1995). *Being-in, being-for, being-with.* Northvale, NJ: Jason Aronson.

National Organization of Nurse Practitioner Faculties. (1995). *Advanced nursing prac-*

tice: Curriculum guidelines and program standards for nurse practitioner education. Washington DC: NONPF.

National Organization of Nurse Practitioner Faculties. (2002). *Domains and core competencies of nurse practitioner practice.* Washington, DC: NONPF.

Nehls, N. (1995). Narrative pedagogy: Rethinking nursing education. *Journal of Nursing Education, 34*(5), 204–210.

Noddings, N. (1984). *Caring: A feminine approach to ethics and moral education.* Berkeley: University of California Press.

Patton, M. Q. (1999). Enhancing the quality and credibility of qualitative analysis. *Health Services Research 34*(5), Part 2, 1189–1208.

Peirce, C. S. (1976). *Collected Papers (Vol. 5).* (C. Hartshorne & P. Weiss, Eds.). Cambridge, MA: Harvard University Press.

Pew Health Professions Commission. (1995). *Critical challenges: Revitalizing the health professions for the twenty-first century.* San Francisco: Pew Health Professions Commission, Center for the Health Professions, University of California.

Polkinghorne, D. (1988). *Narrative knowing and the human sciences.* Albany, NY: State University Press of New York.

Ricouer, P. (1985). History as narrative and practice. *Philosophy Today* (Fall), 213–222. Cited in Anthony Paul Kerby, *Narrative and the self.* (1991). Bloomington: Indiana University Press.

Riessman, C. K. (1993). *Narrative analysis.* Newbury Park, CA: Sage.

Rorty, R. (1999). *Philosophy and social hope.* New York: Penguin.

Sandelowski, M. (2000). Whatever happened to qualitative description? *Research in Nursing & Health, 23,* (4) 334–340.

Schön, D. (1983). *The reflective practitioner: How professionals think in action.* New York: Basic Books.

Schwandt, T. A. (1996). Farewell to criteriology. *Qualitative Inquiry, 2*(1), 58–72.

Swenson, M. M., & Sims, S. L. (2000). Toward a narrative-centered curriculum for nurse practitioners. *Journal of Nursing Education, 39*(3), 109–115.

van Manen, M. (1991). *The tact of teaching: The meaning of pedagogical thoughtfulness.* Albany, NY: State University Press of New York Press.

White, H. (1981). The value of narrativity in the representation of reality. In W. J. T. Mitchell (Ed.), *On narrative.* Chicago: University of Chicago Press.

Young, P. K., & Diekelmann, N. (2002). Learning to lecture: Exploring the skills and strategies of new teachers in nursing education. *Journal of Nursing Education.*

4

Critical Resistance Pathways
Overcoming Oppression in Nursing Education

Rosemary A. McEldowney

My interest in exploring the practices of resisting and accommodating oppression in nursing and nursing education arose from my nursing experiences. In 1995, I explored how nurse educators resisted oppression and, subsequently, I developed the concept of a critical resistance pathway (CRP). The CRP represents a course of action, direction, passage, or journey over time. The journey down the CRP often begins with a felt dis-ease or awareness that includes an understanding of different resistances, such as oppositional or dialectical resistance. Seven markers guide the nurse's journey on the CRP. These markers have emerged from a critique of the literature, theories of resistance, and my autobiographical accounts. The CRP is not finite, fixed, or immutable, but holds open the possibility for others to consider similar or different pathways on which they may journey. To be effective, a CRP should shift us from oppressing or being oppressed to critically resisting oppression. It is intended to be emancipatory, because "resisting," "accommodating," and "enacting" are all lived experiences that can liberate us from oppression.

This chapter presents critical resistance in nursing education as a model of intellectual and critical scholarship and discusses the markers for change that emerged from my literature review and narrative exemplars. A compelling reason for sharing narrative exemplars is that they may encourage other nurse educators to share their stories. Diekelmann (1993) argues, "telling stories publicly is political, critical, and transformative" (p. 6). By telling these stories, I will be able to illuminate the CRP all the more compellingly. I have chosen to give "voice" to my story, so that in naming the multiplicity of our oppressions (racism, sexism, classism) we may discover connections among us and ways to resist and transform our oppressions. If we remain silent, the cycle of oppression will continue to isolate us, cause us pain, and prevent recognition of, or giving value to, our diversity. But, what is "critical resistance"?

Background

Critical resistance is a dynamic process intended to bring about social change. It is a knowing political act—action-oriented, creative, visionary, inclusive, transformative, and empowering. Critical resistance implies taking action to transform the status quo. It is grounded in the struggles of everyday life, struggles to make the personal political, just like feminist theory and the women's movement are concerned both with the struggles of everyday life and the struggle to make the personal political (Boler, 1999; Lather, 1991; Middleton, 1993; Weiler, 1988). Critical resistance in nursing education seeks to counter discourses of domination and recognizes that agency is part of the cycle of resistance and accommodation. Not all types of resistance—for example, dialectic and oppositional resistance—necessarily empower nurse educators or their students. Dialectic resistance occurs when an individual or group recognizes that oppression exists, but through their own volition (agency) decide (consciously) to reject the potential for social change. Instead, they accommodate their oppressive circumstances (Jones, 1991; McFadden, 1995; McRobbie, 1978; Willis, 1977). Oppositional resistance occurs when the desire is to do no more than get a reaction out of the oppressor. This may be manifested in anti-social actions, such as disruptive and distracting, or passive and silent, behaviors (Munns & McFadden, 2000).

Unlike dialectic and oppositional resistance, critical resistance challenges the status quo and counters entrenched patterns of oppression. The critical resister is an active agent who contests hegemonic structures and transforms oppressive power relations. Critical resistance is the catalyst that can break the cycle of interlocking oppressions. It is a pathway that unites resisters and sustains commitments to overcome racism, sexism, and classism. It is about "walking the talk." It arises from critical reflection and action (praxis). On this pathway, "knowing" and "doing" are synchronous and are given expression in organized political resistance. The ability to recognize discourses of dominance and to critique the contradictory positions in which nurse educators are placed in relation to patriarchy provides a basis for critical resistance.

Methodology

The method used in this research involves re-presenting my life story as a way of remembering, reflecting on, and relating significant past events. As a method of narrative inquiry in nursing research, storytelling's momentum has increased. Several nurse academics and researchers have positioned storytelling as an integral aspect of interpretive scholarship in research, practice, and education (Diekelmann, 1993, 1995, 2001; Emden, 1998; Frid, Ohlen & Bergbom, 2000; Ironside, 2001; Koch, 1998; Sandelowski, 1991). In traveling the CRP, one embraces empowering research methodologies with a feminist perspective, methodologies that enable one to participate in revealing false consciousness and in revealing how false consciousness shapes and is shaped by one's experiences.

Focusing the Issues

Early in my research journey, I undertook a life-history project with five feminist nurse educators. It helped me focus on the issues I wished to question and critique. I identified several questions that needed answers. For example: How do nurses and nurse educators remain oppressed? And, if they know they are oppressed, why don't they do something about it? If they do not do something, they continue to "live a lie" and reproduce a system of oppression. After reading the literature on nurses' oppression, I shifted focus and began exploring how nurse educators might resist oppression and break the pattern. I also identified ideas that informed my thinking on the links between feminism and antiracism. I noted, too, that nurse educators who identified themselves as feminists were able to analyze and critique their position in relation to power and their position as active agents in countering hegemony (McEldowney, 1992).

To answer the question "How can nurse educators resist oppression?" I had to establish that nurses and nurse educators are indeed an oppressed group. Drawing on the literature, I explored the historical and structural factors that give rise to and maintain nurses' oppression.

I found evidence that nurses are identified as an oppressed group (Battersby & Hemmings, 1990; Bent, 1993; Bevis & Watson, 1989; Boutain, 1999; David, 2000; Duffy, 1995; Glass, 1997; Kleffel, 1991; Kuokkanen & Leino-Kilpi, 2000; Lee & Saeed, 2001; Rather, 1994; Roberts, 1983, 1997, 2000; Ruffing-Rahal, 1992; Scarry, 1999; Skillings, 1992; Varcoe, 1996; Watson, 1990).

Resistance Theories

I also explored the literature on theories of resistance in education and nursing to establish how individuals or groups resist or accommodate oppression (Apple, 1993; Berlak, 1989; Cleary, 2001; Ellsworth, 1989; Fletcher, 2000; Freire, 1972, 1973; Gewirtz, 1991; Giroux, 1983; Harden, 1996; Jones, 1991; Keddy, 1995; Lather, 1991; Lewis, 1990; McFadden, 1995; McRobbie, 1978; Munns & McFadden, 2000; Pelissier, 1992; Popkewitz & Fendler, 1999; Tatum, 1992; Titus, 2000; Weiler, 1988; Willis, 1977). Keddy (1995) refers to registered nurses enrolled in a baccalaureate nursing program who resisted a feminist critique of nursing. However, she does not address the notion of accommodation. Varcoe (1996), Boutain (1999) and Abrums and Leppa (2001) do offer a critique of the interlocking oppressions of race, gender, and class in nursing. Most of the literature on resistance emerged from theories of resistance related to education, significantly Willis (1977), Apple (1993) and Giroux (1983). The literature search involved the following databases: Cumulative Index of Nursing and Allied Health Literature (CINAHL), Educational Resources Information Center (ERIC), Sociological Abstracts (SOCIOABS), and Studies on Women and Gender Abstracts (SWA).

Critical Feminist Perspective

Many feminist educators offer a critical feminist perspective on schooling, teaching, and learning that addresses issues of social justice, praxis, context, agency, individual voice, and difference (Arnot & Weiler, 1993; Ellsworth, 1989, 1997; Gore, 1993; hooks, 1984, 1995, 2000; Keddy, 1995; Lather, 1991; Luke & Gore, 1992; Middleton, 1993; Munro, 1998; Ng, Staton, & Scane, 1995; Titus, 2000; Weiler, 1988). Their concern is with the lack of critique and analysis of gender and "otherness" by resistance theorists such as Willis (1977) who critique from their ideological and ethnocentric positions as white males within the dominant paradigm. Their concern also arises from a fear of universalism "that silences the voices of all those other than the dominant group" (Warnke, 1993, p. 81).

Gender oppression is no longer the primary issue in feminist politics. It is now a time of multiple contested oppressions. Feminism can also no longer focus on a common unifying oppression or strive for universal emancipation (Boutain, 1999; Cleary, 2001; hooks, 1995; Varcoe, 1996; Yeatman, 1993; Young, 1990). In cultural safety education programs in New Zealand, nurse educators and students now explore dominant and marginalized voices in relation to gender, race and class.[1] As a critical resister, I need to consider my position within emancipatory politics as a white, middle-class woman, otherwise I risk reproducing the dominant ideology through cultural imperialism. As a member of the dominant class in relation to Maori,[2] I am in a privileged position. Different forms of oppression in our society overlap because they arise from the same social structures. As hooks (1984) suggests, "racism is fundamentally a feminist issue because it is so inter-connected with sexist oppression" (p. 51).

Underlying the theoretical approach outlined by critical feminist educators is a commitment to social change that goes beyond equality of access. This approach seeks to reestablish a belief in the need to continue "the struggle for social justice [in terms of class, race, and gender], even within increasingly hostile political environments" (Arnot & Weiler, 1993, p. 3). Critical feminist educators acknowledge the need to theorize oppression and resistance in a way that critiques the construction of difference and "otherness," and that explores the complexities within the three interlocking oppressions. They have also been influenced by the Gramscian notion of hegemony, which seeks to explain how powerful and dominant groups in society maintain social and political control. The dominant view is accepted as common sense and part of the natural order by those who are subordinated to it. Gramsci (1971) asserts that one's consciousness is influenced not only by hegemonic ideas but also by a composite of historical, social, political, and economic forces; visions about the future; and self-reflection and critique. He names this complex consciousness "common sense."

Like resistance and accommodation, hegemony can never be wholly vanquished and is constantly present as individuals contest hegemonic control. According to Weiler (cited in Arnot & Weiler, 1993) the "hegemonic vision glorifies competition and privatization," thereby positioning institutions in thrall to those outside the possibility "of full participation in a democratic society" (p. 215). Because of the emphasis on competition and privatization in the fields of health and education, Weiler contends that a Gramscian perspective is particularly relevant to them. Health and education institutions are hegemonic structures that uphold the ideas, values, and beliefs of dominant groups. These are embedded in the consciousness of the people who work in these institutions. As agents of their own resistance and accommodation, nurses and nurse educators can penetrate these hegemonic structures and transform them.

As nurse educators, we need to move beyond the idea that the mere reproduction of resistance is enough to counter oppressive beliefs and practices within the institution and accept that agency also implies a more critical and politicized work that takes the form of conscious collective opposition (which could include accommodation). Critical resisters make their own position on sexism, classism, and racism overt and render the accepted knowledge of the dominant group problematic.

The Autobiographical Element

Because there was no indigenous material to use as a theoretical basis for how nurse educators resist or accommodate oppression, I decided to tell my own stories. By sharing my stories, the knowledge produced by the unique experiences of my life is preserved and extended. Hearing or reading my stories may help other nurse educators remember their own experiences and forge connections among us. Autobiography (self-narrative) was acknowledged as a research method as far back as the 1920s (Ribbens, 1993). An element of autobiography pervades qualitative research, particularly research in the field of narrative inquiry, because both researchers and participants bring personal experience, feelings, and emotions to the research process (Baisnée, 1997; Brettell, 1997; Church, 1995; Clandinin & Connelly, 2000; Clements, 1999; Cortazzi, 1993; Denzin, 1989; Denzin & Lincoln, 1998; Ellis & Flaherty, 1992; Johnstone, 1999; Richardson, 1998). Johnstone (1999) contends that autobiography is underused in nursing research. It has the potential to contribute to nursing inquiry and knowledge by presenting lived experience as a way to "advance theoretical understanding of the human condition and commonalities in existential human experiences" (p. 136). Clandinin and Connelly (in Denzin & Lincoln,

1998) say that autobiography is an account of particular life experiences, retold and re-presented as "a life as lived" or as the "lived experience." They also suggest that writing about the self amounts to "a particular re-construction of an individual's narrative" that is always open to other reconstructions (p. 167). The act of writing may occur in the present, but autobiographical accounts about that which is past are reflections recalled from memory. Cortazzi (1993) suggests that the autobiographical process is about "reflection upon reflection" (p. 13).

My autobiographical accounts serve as narrative exemplars that provide the reader with an opportunity to engage in the story and in its analysis and interpretation. By providing explicated texts, "common practices and shared experiences" may be recognized. Further "an increased understanding of the meaning and significance of these explicated experiences" can be generated via critical interpretation (Diekelmann, 2001, p. 58).

I adapted the phases of heuristic research described by Moustakas (1990) to write the narrative exemplars and to develop the CRP. Moustakas lists six phases in heuristic research design: initial engagement, immersion, incubation, illumination, explication, and creative synthesis. This approach requires the "researcher as subject" to immerse herself fully in the experience and to engage in reflexivity and critical self-reflection. Moustakas (1990) claims that heuristic research methods are "open-ended," that there is "no exclusive list" of phases one must go through in heuristic investigation and "each research process unfolds in its own way" (p. 43). I ultimately selected four phases to help my research process: immersion, incubation, illumination, and creative synthesis.

During the immersion phase I became deeply involved in thinking about my most significant experiences in resisting and accommodating oppression. This period of deep introspection, from which I generated the raw data for the research, occupied many sleeping, dreaming, and waking moments. This data included events as experienced (the context, other people involved, emotions evoked, responses, and strategies) and self-dialogue. There was a recursive aspect to this self-dialogue as I asked myself questions such as: What made me conscious of oppression in nursing and education? How have I chosen to resist or accommodate that oppression? Is this an accurate account of what happened? Do the exemplars represent my experiences of resistance to, or accommodation of, oppression in nursing practice and education?

The next phase (incubation) involved "letting the draft exemplars sit" and rereading the literature on resistance theory and oppression. An update of the literature search was also required to locate texts, theses, and journal articles that had appeared since I had presented my master's thesis in 1995.

The third phase was one of illumination. Moustakas (1990) says this occurs when there is "a breakthrough into conscious awareness of qualities and a clustering of qualities into themes inherent in the question [or topic]" (p. 29). Illumination occurred for me when I became aware of some key qualities that could serve as markers of the journey on a CRP and of connections among experiences in my everyday life out of which themes might emerge that could contribute to development of a CRP. I also looked for markers and connections in the literature on resistance theories and oppression that could contribute to the pathway.

Finally, creative synthesis entailed writing the narrative exemplars and critically appropriating fragments of theory to illuminate and interpret the experiences. This phase of the process was time-consuming as I wrote and rewrote the exemplars to ensure that they would resonate with readers. Resonance is important to maintaining rigor in storytelling as a research method. It encompasses the ideas of credibility and trustworthiness, and involves creating stories that "ring true" with the reader (Guba & Lincoln, 1989; Hatch & Wisniewski, 1995; Koch & Harrington, 1998).

The seven markers that emerged from this four-phase process were: *breaking the silence, agency, underground movement, other ways of knowing and being, feminism and antiracism, power with/within, and continuity and connection.* The markers represent what I consider are needed to break the cycle of interlocking oppressions. They will continue to evolve, as will my position as a critical resister.

Narrative Exemplars

What made me conscious of oppression in nursing and education? How have I chosen to resist or accommodate that oppression? Answers to these questions are to be found in my gradual move to feminism and in important experiences in both my personal and working life. These turning points or transformations acquired significance when I became critically aware of how certain social and political practices were organized and maintained. Critical awareness and understanding has become the basis of my social and political action. My narrative exemplars represent significant experiences from the 1960s to the late 1990s.

My nursing journey began as a student in a regional hospital in New Zealand with 26 other young women. Three and a half years later only 12 of us graduated. Why did some stay and why did others leave? To become registered nurses, we had to accommodate the bureaucracy by conforming or compromising. In those days I did not know about oppression. However, I had an underlying feeling that some things were not right. Attempts to oppose authority usually elicited a punitive response (often verbal abuse) from the ward sister.[3] One such experience still remains clear in my mind because on reflection it taught me to respond—to give voice to my anger by *breaking the silence.*

One day I was making beds in the women's surgical ward. The ward sister and assistant matron[4] came and stood at the end of the bed. The ward sister began to speak about me in the third person as though I did not exist. She made derogatory remarks about my nursing practice saying that I was slow and was not okay as a nurse. Yet I was considered by the nursing tutors, my peers, other registered nurses, and doctors to be one of the brightest and most competent nursing students. At the time I was also active in the student nurses association and had been stopped in the main hospital corridor by the matron and told that I had far too much influence over the younger nurses.

I finished making the bed and remember the humiliation and pain from her hurtful remarks. The assistant matron didn't stop her. I remember the tears and the feeling of anger and resentment welling up inside me. Realizing that I would say something that I might regret, I walked out of the ward and said that I would not be coming back. I was asked to go to the student health clinic. There I talked to the medical officer about what had occurred. I said that I refused to work anymore on the same ward as the ward sister as she frequently criticized my work, kept me on duty over duty hours, and abused me verbally. She only spoke nicely to the doctors or senior nursing staff. Her behavior was the same with most students. My peers who had spent time on the ward had all come off duty in tears because of her behavior toward them. I suggested to the medical officer that because of her behavior she was not suited to the position of ward sister.

Consequently, I was sent to another ward, but not before my mental state had been questioned. The doctor considered me to be the one with the problem because I was angry and tearful. However, he did listen to my account of what had happened and I did get to move. I never checked to find out if the doctor ever spoke with the ward sister.

Reflecting on this event, I realized that what I had experienced was horizontal hostility. Horizontal hostility is intergroup conflict that occurs because of lack of self-esteem, lack of autonomy, fear of success, divisiveness, lack of participation in professional organizations, and ineffective leadership (Duffy, 1995; Glass, 1997; Roberts, 1983, 2000). It is manifested in behaviors such as criticism, scapegoating, infighting, and bullying. At the time, I did not know to label this behavior as horizontal hostility or that this behavior stemmed from oppression among nurses. I also reflected on whether the ward sister and assistant matron behaved the way they did because of their own oppression and inability to resist the dominant ideology in the institution. With *"the tears and the feeling of anger and resentment welling up inside me,"* I, however, chose instead to become an active agent in my own resistance and refused to accommodate the horizontal hostility toward me. Although the doctor thought I might have a problem because I was angry and tearful, he *listened* to me, and I was given the opportunity to move to another area of practice. I felt that I had been *heard* and that my voice did make a difference. My resistance *(breaking the silence)* was a first step on the CRP.

Institutions we grew up in and still work in have traditionally silenced women's voices (Buresh & Gordon, 2000; Glass, 1994,1998; Parker & Gardiner, 1992). Breaking silence and giving voice to our lived experiences through stories informs the theory and practice of critical resistance. We need to step out of line, stop obeying, stop complying, refuse to keep silent, refuse to lie, and refuse to not know what is going on. Nurses are silenced within education and health institutions because the dominant culture minimizes our needs and interests. We need to tell our stories as an act of resistance and not lessen their impact or conceal them to make them more acceptable and inoffensive (Banks-Wallace, 1998). Our collective stories then become more politically significant as we identify our lived experiences of subordination to patriarchal hegemony. Naming our oppressions breaks the silence.

To break my silence, I needed to bring forth a sense of *agency*. Agency makes possible a political commitment to empowerment and social transformation (Freire, 1972; Lather, 1991; McFadden, 1995; Weiler, 1988). Agency is another vital marker on the CRP. These two markers, breaking the silence and agency, recur and co-occur in my other exemplars. Perhaps it was this sense of agency and breaking the silence that enabled me to complete my training.

Working Underground

Another important marker on my CRP—*underground movement*—surfaced when I began work in psychiatric (mental health) nursing. The underlying reason why many women were admitted to the psychiatric unit, which was sexual, physical, or emotional abuse, was seldom acknowledged. One woman's experience stands out:

On an afternoon shift in the psychiatric unit of a city hospital, I was asked to admit a woman called Jane who had been diagnosed as being depressed. She had already attempted to kill herself a few days earlier by running her car off the road. I was asked to do an initial nursing assessment. The doctor had done a physical assessment and checked her mental state, but no details were given about the reason for her depression and suicide attempt.

During my conversation with Jane she told me that she had been married to a successful businessman and had four children. Her husband had left her recently after 20 years of marriage. Jane also disclosed that he had physically abused her at times, but she continued to love him and pretended that their marriage was fine. When I checked out about the attempted suicide she said that running the car off the road was a sudden half-hearted attempt to end it all because she felt angry and bereft that her husband had deserted her.

For several days, Jane talked about her life and her role as a mother and wife. She did not want to stay in the unit. She did not consider herself seriously depressed and wanted to return home to her children. She said that the doctor had not talked with her about why she had been diagnosed with depression or why she was prescribed antidepressants. He was adamant that she stay in the unit for at least two weeks.

I found that the institutional and medical "rules" conflicted with my belief about what Jane had shared as being important for her at this time. Together Jane and I negotiated a way for her to stay safe and accommodate the system. We organized for her to go home each day to be with her children. A close friend would come and pick her up in the afternoon (following the doctor's round) and bring her back after a few hours. The friend was also able to keep Jane safe and always kept in touch during this time. We often talked about how it was like working undercover as part of an underground movement.

So, I worked in two worlds. On one hand, I nursed Jane in a way that was in line with the medical diagnosis she had received because that was the system and I did not want to compromise her position. On the other hand, I acknowledged the caring and healing aspect of the nurse's role by recognizing and acknowledging Jane's experiences. Hutchinson (1990) describes this process as *responsible subversion—* bending the rules in the best interests of the patient. I bent the rules for Jane by negotiating *a way for her to stay safe and accommodate the system.*

Women like Jane often carry invisible wounds that reflect social and political injustices. These wounds are not always acknowledged by medical and nursing staff. Jane's doctor *had not talked with her about why she had been diagnosed with depression or why she was prescribed antidepressants. He was adamant that she stay in the unit for at least two weeks.* If women patients do not conform to the male-defined norm for a woman, then medical staff often diagnose (label) them as having depression, schizophrenia, or personality disorders. Chesler (1989) contends that very few women admitted to a psychiatric unit have a mental disturbance. Instead, they are responding to the oppressions in their lives. Steen (1991) asserts, "oppression of women on the basis of gender as well as of class and race is the basis for the conflicts, low self-esteem, and powerlessness reported by many women who seek therapy" (p. 366).

Jane's experiences needed to be validated. It was a time to break the silence, to make visible the invisible, and to identify and value the connectedness with or intuitive knowing about women's worlds that arose from her stories. I often feel that I am working in an underground movement with women to try and resist and overcome their medicalization. Rich (1979) describes an underground life of women that has existed for centuries. Maintaining an underground movement enables women to keep themselves safe, to reflect, and to preserve energy. Although they may appear exclusive, underground movements offer an opportunity for all women. We go within our deep female psyches to create spaces wherein our visions and creativity can emerge, and to restore our energies and reflect on the daily paradoxes in our lives (Estes, 1992).

Women as nurses inhabit a similar world to that of many of their patients. As workers, and as patients, we occupy both hierarchical and oppressive social spaces. Struggling with the dominant paradigm and living in silence, we hide behind a mask, wishing to be accepted and acknowledged by those in power. "Hidden transcripts," or forms of resistance that nurses and their women patients engage in away from the eyes and ears of the dominant group help keep them safer (Pelissier, 1992). Through Jane, I became involved in the collective struggle with patients to claim their voices. I have often revisited the idea of two worlds in which nurses and patients move, an external world, on the one hand, of authority and control where there is separation of mind and body and an internal world, on the other, of self-integrity and intuition where there is *connection and continuity* and *other ways of knowing and being* (Baker & Diekelmann, 1994; Diekelmann & Diekelmann, forthcoming; Estes, 1992; Belenky, Clinchy, Goldberger, & Tarule, 1986; Glass, 1997, 1998; Ironside, 2001; Starhawk, 1990).

Other Ways of Knowing and Being

During the 1970s the second wave of feminism arrived and with it *other ways of knowing and being*—another CRP marker. As a wife and mother, I felt that something was happening to unsilence women. I began to question women's roles in the family and society. I wanted to extend my knowledge, so I enrolled at university as an extramural (distance) student. I spent time reading, thinking, and reflecting about the changes that were going on. University courses held during vacation times enabled extramural students (women, wives, and mothers) to share stories. Although I wasn't able to name it at the time, I was coming to a critical consciousness of my being in the world. Freire (1972, 1973) named this process *conscientization*—when teachers and students become active agents or subjects who construct and reconstruct the meaning of their lives. Nurse educators who critically resist are aware that they (and their students) are historically situated subjects with conflicting and competing attitudes about race, gender, and class. During this time I also returned to full-time work as a nurse educator in a hospital-based program. One of my roles was preparing second-year students to work in surgical nursing. Other health professionals shared their knowledge. One demonstrated the need for another CRP marker—*power with/within*:

During a study week I asked a surgeon to talk about his management of cancer patients. He said he never told terminal cancer patients what the outcome was. He always talked as if they were never going to die. I could not believe this and asked him why? He responded, "Well, would you want to know?" He probably had his reasons, but ultimately he excluded the patient from knowing. Later, I became involved in working with a community nurse who was caring for one of the surgeon's patients who had cancer with a poor prognosis. The patient and his wife were my neighbors. He had been discharged not knowing his true position. The surgeon had told him to put on a bit more weight, so that he (the surgeon) could operate and repair a hernia that had been troubling the patient. One day I met the community nurse who had been visiting Mr. Brown (not his real name). Mrs. Brown was distressed because Mr. Brown was getting worse and she couldn't understand why. The nurse and I talked about it and she told Mr. and Mrs. Brown about Mr. Brown's diagnosis and prognosis. The Browns were so relieved because it meant they could plan for the future and settle their affairs. They were also angry with the surgeon for withholding the information and giving them false hope. As a result of this experience, I worked with a group of nurses, doctors, and church ministers to run lunchtime seminars on dying, grief, and loss for all hospital staff. It was the first time a collective response was initiated among health professionals in that small provincial hospital. The seminars were well attended.

The example of the Browns made me realize that doctors can end up rendering their patients dependent on their judgment in their effort to protect them, and thereby control knowledge and power (Bunkle, 1992; White, 1999). Yet patients also contribute to medical knowledge and power through their lived experiences of illness. The withholding of information from the Browns is an example of how a doctor can appeal to the idea that the doctor knows best in order to control the patient

and deny him his personal experience of illness (White, 1999). This excluded the Browns from knowing and being able to decide for themselves what future arrangements they might need to make because of
Mr Brown's poor prognosis. Recently, changes in the law have given
healthcare consumers a more powerful voice.[5]

The Vulnerable Patient

Another time of transformation in my life brought the issue of accommodating oppression starkly into view. It highlighted a situation of
critical resistance within accommodation—that is, a situation in which
one could be more effective by not pushing the boundaries.

*I was admitted to hospital with a life-threatening condition, which
placed me in a position of dependency on medical and nursing staff. I
was also marginalized as a patient because of my position as a nurse
educator and because I expressed my feelings about being ignored or not
having care negotiated with me. Nursing and medical staff and students
tended to avoid me, possibly due to embarrassment or because they assumed that as a nurse I knew enough about the system to not require
care or explanation. I recall moments of anger and resistance at being
discounted. The morning after I had been to the operating room a staff
nurse came into the room with breakfast. I had an intravenous infusion
in my left arm and an abdominal wound that made it very difficult to
move. The staff nurse placed my tray on a table some distance away
from my bed and told me to get up. She did not offer any assistance.
When I asked to have the tray given to me in bed, she replied that "all
patients get up for breakfast in this ward, and you are no exception." I
protested because it was painful and awkward for me to sit at a table.
She would not give me the tray, so I went without breakfast. I felt angry
about her response and asked to talk to the charge nurse of the ward
who told me not to create trouble. Because I was in a vulnerable position
due to my physical and mental condition, I ended up accommodating
the situation in order to complete my stay in the ward with as minimal
resistance as possible.*

The staff nurse was going to follow the rules regardless of what might
be happening for me as a patient—*"all patients get up for breakfast in
this ward, and you are no exception."* What happened to me also made
me question how often patients accommodate a situation because they

are vulnerable. Yet nurses should be able to adapt to the needs of the client. They do not need to remain rule-driven and powerless in their daily practice. They do not need to resist knowing about what other possibilities exist. Nor do they need to place patients in a subordinate and powerless position. On reflection, I saw that *my anger and resistance at being discounted* and being silenced became a catalyst for confronting the "silencing concretely" (Lewis & Simon, 1986, p. 465). This experience reinforced my resolve to support patients by listening to what was happening for them.

The Greatest Challenge

My greatest challenge as a critical resister and a nurse leader occurred after I was appointed dean of a nursing school. It coincided with the introduction of cultural safety into the national undergraduate nursing program. The ten years before my appointment was a time of personal transformation. As a conscientized Pakeha[6] nurse educator belonging to the dominant culture, I frequently asked myself the following question: If I felt marginalized and oppressed as a woman and nurse, then how did Maori feel? Two events transformed my views on racism in New Zealand. First was a tour by a whites-only South African rugby football team.[7] Second was a Maori student nurses' hui (gathering) at a place called Ratana. Both brought into focus another CRP marker—the links between *feminism and antiracism*.

I attended the Ratana hui as an observer—to support Maori students and to listen. At the hui I heard the voices of Maori students and registered nurses sharing their concerns and feelings about marginalization within nursing education and as recipients of healthcare. Prominent Maori (doctors, nurses, educators, and politicians) spoke of the need for them to determine their own health and education outcomes. Maori students asked for education that would better suit their needs and prepare them for nursing. Three other Pakeha feminist nurse educators attended the hui with me. We resolved to address the issues raised—such as recognizing differences in the learning needs of Maori students, creating a safer learning environment, and including a Maori health perspective within the curriculum. As I became aware of issues of marginality and inequalities of access for women and Maori to power and knowledge, I began to make connections between feminism and antiracism. The five feminist nurse educators I interviewed for the life-history project also acknowledged this connection. They considered that feminism and anti-racism were interrelated because both women and Maori were oppressed by patriarchal domination in healthcare and education.

As a Pakeha feminist nurse educator, I recognize that oppression is different for Maori and Pakeha women. Pakeha feminists are not able to articulate their issues within a Maori cultural framework as they are part of the dominant culture. I need to analyze power relations and avoid becoming another oppressive agent in relation to Maori women. Oppression arises from, and colonization is the result of, dominant patriarchal Pakeha structures of which I am a part (Smith, 1993). Maori women's struggles are their own, not an adjunct of Pakeha women's struggles. A Maori nurse educator colleague explains: "We do not need rescuing. We want to have the opportunity to meet our own needs in our own way. What we do want is your support to work alongside us, not against us" (Fox, 1994, foreword). My position now on antiracism is that I am committed to supporting Maori women in their struggle for self-determination by critiquing the dominant forms of knowledge and the structures that oppress Maori.

Cultural Safety Mandate

When cultural safety was introduced into New Zealand nursing in 1992, it gave educators and practitioners the mandate to address issues of inequity in education and health for Maori. It also provides a focus for the CRP markers of agency, breaking the silence, other ways of knowing and being, feminism and antiracism, and power with/within. Cultural safety education, the basis of which is attitude and behavioral change, involves critical analysis of the discourses of dominance, such as Western dualism, oppression, colonization, and power. It explores personal and institutional power relationships and the culture of poverty, and urges the surrender of power and control by the dominant culture (Ramsden, 1992).

However, at the time the cultural safety programs were introduced New Right ideologues were not prepared to give up power without a struggle. In the ensuing public debate, cultural safety became a political scapegoat for those who wished to challenge its development. Those espousing hegemonic ideologies positioned those working to overcome the oppressions of race, gender, and class as being "politically correct." The cries of political correctness came from those who wished to provide "a convenient excuse to silence dissent or criticism of the status quo" (Weiler, 1993, p. 221). The cultural safety course, as a critical pedagogy, challenges the underlying power of the status quo and critiques sociopolitical and economic policies. Together, teacher and student constantly negotiate, impose, and resist meaning according to their own subjectivities. The classroom discourse associated with cultural safety is never neutral, but is contextually situated in the socially and historically defined present. Questions are constantly asked, such as: What is happening here? Why are things the way they are? Who gets to speak? Who speaks for whom? Who has the power?

It was important for both nurse educators and students to critique the media's coverage of the cultural safety debate—for example, its coverage of opposition to the program by some students and educators. The media is subject to hegemonic influence that reinforces the status quo, and so it was also important to identify the prevailing discourses, such as institutional power, oppression, and resistance. Rather than close the debate down, we chose to keep the process open so that different viewpoints, including resistance to cultural safety, could be voiced. It was also a time of connection and continuity between those educators who were involved in teaching cultural safety courses and colleagues who supported them. The process of dialogue and critical self-reflection through emancipatory discourse enabled us to see ourselves as active agents in challenging and changing our daily-lived experiences.

Antiracism Education

Antiracism education, a part of the cultural safety program, is an example of a critical pedagogy that I have been involved in. As an educator in cultural safety, I have observed student resistance to knowing about personal and structural racism.

Antiracism education involves attitude change, which can be sensitive, emotional, and painful. Students express feelings that range from anger and hostility to sadness and disbelief. Because of discomfort and dissonance, it is inevitable that resistance will occur. I recall some examples of students' verbal responses, which indicate resistance:

"I'm not racist, but . . ."

"How come no one ever told us this before?"

"Why are you trying to make me feel guilty for something I didn't do?"

"There's nothing I can do. I don't have the power."

Students often worry about other people's feelings and leave things unsaid. Also, students from minority or subordinate groups, such as Maori, may not feel safe disclosing their feelings about racism. One helpful process was to work with a colleague rather than alone to ensure continuity and connection and to keep safe. We shared stories of how we came to understand issues of race, gender, and class. It is important to facilitate a process that is respectful of all students regardless of how and where they are positioned. For example, Maori students were not present when issues of racism were discussed with Pakeha students.

Working with racism can be both powerful and isolating. Powerful, because once we become conscientized and acknowledge responsibility for personal and structural racism we can take action to address it. Isolating, because Pakeha can find themselves no longer "fitting into their own cultural settings as well as they once did" (Kirton, 1997, p. 139). Students tend to resist confronting racism because they stand in multiple and contradictory positions in relation to their own experiences of it. Often these positions coincide with the discursive practices of the dominant culture. A Pakeha student's position on race and racism, for example, may reflect that of family members, friends, and colleagues who have not critiqued issues of race and who may also challenge the student's developing knowledge in the interests of maintaining the status quo. Students may also experience tension in the classroom because of their perceptions of caring and nurturing, which are historically and socially constructed, and the desire to maintain existing relations. They may worry about others' feelings and want to rescue them from discomfort, or they may leave their ideas unsaid to protect their colleagues, friends and themselves from confrontation.

When a student offers a critique of different histories the exercise reveals her or his ability to draw on knowledge in order to affirm her or his own identity. Antiracism educators need to search for the emancipatory and liberatory elements that may underpin resistance, render them visible, and develop them as objects of debate and political analysis. Being aware of student responses such as: *"I'm not racist, but . . . ,"* enables the nurse educator to recognize student resistance.

Several antiracist educators have written about resistance to knowing about racism (Abrums & Leppa, 2001; Derman-Sparks & Phillips, 1997; hooks, 1995; Tatum, 1992). Tatum identifies three major barriers to learning about race and racism. First, it is difficult to have a frank discussion of race and racism in racially mixed groups. Second, many students have been socialized into thinking that theirs is a fair and just society (i.e., the myth of meritocracy). Third, many white students deny any personal prejudice and discrimination. What frequently happens in the classroom is a collision of developmental processes relating to racial identity development for black and white students. Tatum argues that working through the stages of racial identity development theory with students undertaking racism awareness programs, serves as a useful journey from racist to antiracist consciousness. It assists black students to shift from rejecting their racial identity to an understanding of who they are in the world and to engaging in antiracist activity. It also assists white students to shift from an ethnocentric position to "naming their racism" and engaging in antiracist activity. Although educational institutions may not change society, antiracism education may create an opportunity for critical resistance to develop. Other ways of knowing and being, which promote social justice and equity, may follow.

Some feminists and feminist educators argue that we need to ensure that our own subject positions do not go unexamined (Ellsworth, 1989; Gore, 1993; Lather, 1991; Lewis, 1990; Luke & Gore, 1992; Middleton, 1993; Nicholson, 1990; D. Smith, 1987). We need to look closely at "how we contribute to dominance in spite of our liberatory intentions" (Lather, 1991, p. 15). It is always possible that efforts to teach in an emancipatory way will end up being oppressive and maintain resistance. For example, feminist educators might be tempted to view a resister as someone infused with false consciousness who cannot see the "light." To overcome this tendency to judge others in this way we need a critical feminist pedagogy that, rather than suppressing the personal, makes "visible to and explore[s] with our students the aspects of our own life histories that impact on our teaching" (Middleton, 1993, p. 17). This involves examining how our personal and pedagogical perspectives are situated within particular historical, social, political, and auto/biographical contexts, and how these perspectives are shaped or restricted by broader power relations (Middleton, 1993). While a critical feminist pedagogy may give "voice" to the experiences of marginalized and oppressed groups, nurse educators (as emancipatory teachers) need to avoid becoming the "masters of truth and justice" imposing their own truths on others (Foucault, 1977, p. 12).

Nurse educators, as critical resisters, need to be conscious of critical education theories and critical feminist theories; be clear about the specific meanings of sexism, racism, and classism; locate themselves within the complex of social relationships as historically constructed and gendered subjects; and act to encourage resistance to oppression. Awareness of gender, race, and class will place nurse educators at the center of transformation and social change and counter the reproduction of oppressions.

Becoming a Critical Resister

So, how might nurse educators achieve the knowledge and insight to become critical resisters? Useful strategies include: networking nationally and locally with other nurse educators who teach cultural safety (e.g., sharing resources and discussing helpful processes), joining politically active groups such as an antiracism coalition or women's network, grounding oneself in one's identity as a nurse and educator, continuing to read and critique literature related to research-based pedagogies, and mentoring or learning from nurse educators who are acknowledged by their colleagues and students as working in an emancipatory way.

For me, being the leader of a nursing school highlighted both personal and theoretical issues of resistance and accommodation. Because of the time and energy I spent as dean in critically resisting an oppressive system, it became important for me to call on all CRP markers. Leadership tasks included managing people, academic matters, and resources and working with colleagues to create an emancipatory vision for nursing, midwifery, and health education. From the outset, I had to withstand critical and personal attacks.

As the "outsider" (the person from outside the organization who got the job), I was marginalized by some who had wanted the dean's job. Because I wished to address issues of power-over (dominance) and violence that were occurring and creating a "culture of silence," various attempts were made to silence and discredit me. At times, I felt an affinity with the witches of the sixteenth and seventeenth centuries, although my oppressors restricted themselves to metaphorically burning me at the stake. For example, allegations were made to senior managers by a male staff member that I was both "mad and bad." Mad, because I was "psychotic, had bouts of depression and had been a patient in a mental hospital and they knew someone who had nursed me." Bad, because I dared to talk about issues of power and politics within the department, including the importance of resisting power-over. These allegations were presented to me by the deputy CEO (chief executive officer), who then proceeded to ask me questions about my mental health because, he said, "I need to make sure that there are no underlying issues here that I don't know about and that could be substantiated." I recall feeling as if I had been "done over." I had a strong desire to walk away and never go back. It took some strong self-talk and calling on the power within to turn around, go back and resist the power-over.

I settled the allegations by taking out a case of defamation and received an apology. Although it was a work-related incident, I received no support from senior management. Male managers tried to keep me in my place—that is, on the periphery with minimal access to power and resources. I thought and interpreted things differently than many of my male senior colleagues. If I resisted or challenged the center of patriarchal power then I was *peripheralized* (Hall, Stevens, & Meleis, 1994, p. 25). I was peripheralized in numerous ways. Key information required to make informed decisions was withheld from me, and decisions were made about nursing and midwifery without consultation with me that I would first find out about in the daily newspaper. I was also peripheralized by the fact that there was no adequate Equal Employment Opportunity (EEO) policy to maintain a safe workplace for women. But with a strong sense of agency, one can challenge hierarchical power. Hall, Stevens, and Meleis (1994) define this as "horizontal power . . . which is exerted by the marginalized in resistance to the hegemony of the center" (p. 28).

For me it was important to break the silence (and denial) evident in the school. This involved opening things up for debate and change. There was a certain element of risk and daring involved, because conflict can be expected whenever there is change. If there is no resistance, then it is unlikely that anything is changing (Starhawk, 1987). One of the reasons my position was challenged owed to my commitment to the cultural safety program. I had to stand my ground with senior management and some nursing staff who continued to resist the idea of analyzing and critiquing our multiple subjectivities in relation to race, gender, and class issues (Weiler, 1988). As I critically resisted, challenged, and made demands of the patriarchal institution, it resisted back. Often I felt betrayed by those who had the power, but who "looked away" (Estes, 1992). It is a mistake to believe that people with power will make it easy for us to bring about change. The journey on the CRP includes a restless to-ing and fro-ing. I recognized the need to accommodate some situations because I could be more effective by remaining in the job than by leaving or being dismissed. This is critical resistance within accommodation.

One positive aspect of critically resisting was the growing awareness of some nurse educator colleagues of the need to open up debate and critique issues of oppression and domination in nursing. Recognition of the CRP markers breaking the silence, other ways of knowing and being, and power with/within was occurring. Staff were beginning to identify power-with and power-within and to critically resist power-over. They were also learning to recognize marginalization. Much of what we do comes from embedded knowledge and the practical knowing of every-day life as women and nurses (Benner, 1984; Diekelmann, 2001) that is not part of the mainstream. Exploring these forms of knowledge through converging conversations, we are able to identify the connections in our lived experiences. It is the everydayness that keeps nursing going and holds it together. As nurse educators, we need to voice our everyday experiences that are silenced in their everydayness (Diekelmann & Diekelmann, in press).

Entrapped by Oppression

After four years of cultural safety education in nursing, the govern-ment bowed to political pressure and undertook a national review. Some nurse educators and students opposed cultural safety, but two key inci-dents caused the politicians to call for a review. The first incident (which occurred in another nursing school) involved a nursing student who challenged a Maori kaumatua (elder) during a session on a marae (meet-ing place) and who subsequently failed her cultural safety course. The second incident (which occurred in our school) involved a nurse educa-tor who was dismissed by the CEO because he chose to air his concerns about cultural safety in the media rather than deal with them in the school. I offered him opportunities to talk about his concerns, but he avoided discussing them with me and other staff members.

The Nursing Council of New Zealand[8] negotiated to undertake the review in the seventeen nursing schools throughout New Zealand. They set up a panel of three. As dean of the school, I was to meet the review panel and arrange for staff and students to meet them, too. The three also met the institute's CEO and the deputy CEO. The CEO had just been appointed from Canada, and so was still coming to terms with cultural safety. Over the next few weeks two of the CRP markers (underground movement and continuity and connection) were to become indispensable.

On the day of the panel's visit to our school I felt apprehensive. I knew that the nurse educator who had been dismissed had arranged a private meeting with the panel, and I was also aware that some of his supporters did not want to go with other staff members to talk with the inquiry team—they claimed they "did not feel safe with their colleagues." He was no longer a member of staff and had taken out a personal grievance case against me and the CEO because of his dismissal.

I met with the inquiry team and discussed development of the cultural safety program including preparation of teaching staff and an overview of the program. Because the dismissed nurse educator's personal grievance case was sub judice, I never talked about him with the panel members.[9]

I was not present for the conversation between the CEO, deputy CEO, and the panel; however, I did join the cultural safety teaching team when they met the panel. One of the things I observed throughout the meeting was that the panel never questioned any comments made by staff—therefore anyone was able to say exactly what they liked without providing any rationale or evidence.

Later, I was called to the CEO's office. When I walked into his office only he and the deputy CEO were present. I sensed that something was wrong. The CEO told me that the inquiry panel had raised issues about my role as dean and my management of the school in relation to cultural safety. The deputy CEO said that he could understand that this would be hard for me to take given all the work I had done for cultural safety and that this would be damaging for me both personally and professionally. The CEO said I was "not to say anything to anyone—just to keep the conversation in-house and between us so as not to damage your reputation." He then suggested that I "take a couple of days to think about this and to reconsider [my] position within the institution" and let him know by Monday what I intended to do.

I felt as if the carpet had been pulled out from underneath me and my reaction was one of overwhelming sadness and anger that without any opportunity for redress, they could lay all the ills of cultural safety on me. I asked if they had anything in writing from the panel and they replied that "no it was verbal feedback." As I felt myself getting more and more angry and felt the tears starting to come I stood up and left the room—fearing that I might say something that might be further used in evidence against me. One of the things that really made me angry was that they had asked me to come with no support person. The process was unfair and unjust. I felt that I had been betrayed by the CEO and deputy CEO on the basis of hearsay and innuendo. I went back to the school and immediately spoke with two colleagues and said, "I think I've just been given the sack because of the cultural safety inquiry." They asked what had happened and we then began the process of organizing a response. The underground movement and network of support was set into motion.

Twenty-four hours later I had been offered the services of a lawyer, the trade union had advised me to write down exactly what happened in the CEO's office, and many staff, students, graduates, cultural safety advisory group members, local Maori and practice colleagues, and other colleagues nationally were asked to submit a statement to the CEO that I had worked to establish a strong cultural safety program and parallel program for Maori and that I needed to continue in my job. I contacted a panel member and asked if they had spoken to the CEO about me in the way he had related it. The panel member responded that they had not.

I was not going to go without a fight. Over the next three weeks the trade union attempted to communicate with the CEO about my situation and to request a meeting to discuss why I had to reconsider my position. The CEO refused to meet with me. I had to continue going to work each day and maintaining a presence for the school while continuing my resistance to the CEO's position.

Eventually I had a meeting with the CEO with trade union people present. He was unable to provide any evidence from the panel in writing and had received an overwhelming show of support from many clinicians, nurse educators, and students that convinced him I needed to stay. I received a verbal and written apology from the CEO and all documentation that he had written was removed from my file.

This story is an example of critically resisting a situation of power-over. The CEO did not handle my case fairly. The way he treated me contravened what was required under legislation and conflicted with what was expected of me in handling employment-related issues with my staff. The supportive network established through the continuity and connection with the community and my understanding of my rights as an employee enabled me to stand my ground and critically resist the power-over of the CEO.

Nurse educators, as historically situated subjects, have their own issues of power, race, gender, and class to consider within a hegemonic education institution. One issue is that our own racist, sexist, and classist beliefs and practices can come between ourselves and our students preventing what Freire (1972) refers to as "dialogic" education. Furthermore, women as nurse educators can be subject to resistance from male colleagues who have a vested interest in maintaining their position of male privilege. As nurse educators, it is essential that we challenge truths imposed on us and take responsibility for our own truths and actions. Refusing to be isolated by building a strong sense of community is a formidable and powerful act of resistance. Power with, or horizontal power as it is defined by Hall, Stevens, and Meleis (1994) "is that which is exerted by the marginalized in resistance to the hegemony of the center" (p. 28). The knowledge that exists at the margins enables oppressed groups, such as nurses, to resist subordination and engage in other transformative possibilities—the CRP markers of breaking the silence, agency, the underground movement, other ways of knowing and being, feminism and antiracism, power with/within, and continuity and connection.

Time for Transformation

Nurse educators who are critical resisters have a vision of a socially just world and are proactive in their attempts to bring about social transformation and liberation. They have a strong sense of social justice in their lives. Critical resisters within an educational institution go through a process of conscientisation that enables them to identify and critically analyze their own position. They are able to identify the institution as a combination of political, personal, and social forces that can either dominate or liberate. Critical resisters also recognize that the competing forces of domination and liberation can, and do, mutually inform each other. Critical resisters identify and create an opening in which to raise social and political issues for debate. They are active agents for social change.

Nurse educators who critically resist are often involved in antiracist activities, but they also address gender and class issues in the classroom. To critically resist, nurse educators need to know themselves—to know who one really is as a result of historical and social processes that have been embedded in one's consciousness. Traditionally, nurses have been separated and alienated from one another, because of their subordinated position within the health care system (Duffy, 1995; Roberts, 1983). Being subordinate has contributed to nurses perceiving themselves as being powerless to bring about change. This position has prevented them from attaining solidarity and collective activism. To teach and nurse effectively, we need to know ourselves. This is what we bring to our teaching and nursing partnerships, and it can be a catalyst for provoking caring and social change. To critically resist, nurse educators need to be conscious of their own subjectivities; by so doing they can affirm and challenge the lived experiences of others.

Nurse educators who are critical resisters experience conflict with students and other nurse educators who are likewise embedded in historically and socially constructed positions and who have incorporated male hegemony into their consciousness. The goals of feminist and antiracist nurse educators are transformative and challenging. This can threaten other nurse educators or those in positions of authority who still cling to traditional pedagogies and hierarchical ways of teaching (Diekelmann, 1995; Ironside, 2001). As a dean I followed through on my commitment to critically resisting sexism, racism, and classism by hiring staff who were also committed to these goals, by providing workshops for ongoing staff development that focused on critiquing racism, sexism, and classism, by team building, and by maintaining a non-hierarchical management structure with shared responsibility. Further, staff are required to attend workshops on the Treaty of Waitangi,[10] negotiated partnership, and cultural safety. My talking about women's and nurses' oppression and racism creates conflict for some staff and students. However, I need to be optimistic and focused, to keep my goals and vision clear, to maintain a feminist and antiracist curriculum, and to believe that people can change. Structural forces may shape and limit my work, but the commitment I have to critical resistance has brought about change.

Discussion

By reflecting on narrative exemplars of resisting and accommodating oppression and identifying markers on the critical resistance pathway, I have further developed a consciousness and awareness of how nurse educators can engender socially critical attitudes and practices. As nurse educators, we are embedded in two cultures—the education institution and nursing practice. This contributes to the paradoxical nature of our work. Nurse educators experience tensions between social structures and individual *agency* while engaged in producing and reproducing a professional nursing culture. Their individual consciousness can be seen to be socially constructed within these institutional contexts where structured power relationships are well established. However, while nurse educators are determined by their historical and social circumstances, they have the capacity to reflect and free themselves from oppression. Nurse educators who critically resist act to critique and transform the social world they inhabit. In this chapter, I have not only addressed issues of patriarchal hegemony, but have moved beyond single oppressions, such as gender oppression. I have described a path by which nurse educators, as critical resisters, can highlight the complexity of social sites where differing raced, classed, and gendered subjectivities come together, but not in isolation from the wider society. For these institutions can mirror the contradictions and tensions in society affected by oppressions and inequalities.

The basis of nurse educators' work as critical resisters is to be aware of contradictions that arise through everyday experiences of power and oppression for our students and us and to value the voices of students and colleagues. If the process fails, the status quo is reproduced in the preservation of a hierarchical power-over relationship between nurse educator and student. However, there are many structural issues that threaten our work as nurse educators, such as economic restraints that affect resources and centralized control of curricula by bureaucracies. We are also seen as functionaries in a technological world where the goal is to produce outputs with quantifiable results. Too often, the measure of our success is how many students graduate. But although the institution may be a site of social reproduction for nursing students, it is also a site where challenges to the dominant ideology can occur. Both nurse educators and students can create and reshape knowledge and values. The classroom can become the site where the discourse of possibility (such as critical resistance) can be constructed (Apple, 1993).

To facilitate student empowering processes, nurse educators themselves must also be empowered. This is where the critique of resistance to, or accommodation of, interlocking oppressions needs to be a priority. If we cannot critically reflect on our own lived experiences of oppression, then we will not be in a position to work critically with students. I have been able to identify some reasons why nurse educators may not critically resist. Individuals may resist in a rebellious or oppositional way that does not lead to critical resistance via ongoing social action (oppositional resistance), or they may resist in a way that supports the dominant ideology and leaves them politically defeated (dialectic resistance). This can occur due to living in ignorance, not even thinking about oppressions, just "getting on with life," or accommodating the status quo.

They may resist, too, because of fear—fear of being exposed as dominant, fear of losing dominance, or fear of power. People may not wish to expose oppression for fear of what might happen if they do speak out. Resistance to knowing about one's own oppression could also be due to "dangerous memories"—a psychological response to our own experiences of internalized oppressions (Berlak, 1989). Or an individual may resist in a way that says, "I know I am oppressed and that racism, sexism, classism exists, but so what? Why should I do anything about it? It won't make a bit of difference."

Another reason why we as nurse educators may resist knowing about our oppression is internalization of patriarchal hegemony through being a woman and nurse that devalues our worth and marginalizes us. We can make choices, but only within the context of existing structures and ideologies that have influenced us from our entrance into society and that have been reinforced through the institutions that we inhabit. In her doctoral research on a critical approach to teaching and learning in nursing, Clare (1991) reveals that nurse educators were not reflexive in the sense of coming to understand what must change to transform oppressive conditions in their work and then acting on that understanding. However, as a result of critical dialogue with the researcher, their subsequent actions were more socially conscious and reflective and the potential for transformative action increased.

Because teaching is valuable political work, we need to free ourselves from the isolation and competition that entraps us. We need to work collectively on creating curricula, relationships, and non-hierarchical work places. This means critiquing oppressions that occur in our daily lives. It will generate conflict, tension, and resistance as I have suggested in my narrative exemplars. However, it must be done if we want to prevent the ongoing reproduction of nurses' oppression. Nurse educators who do not critique their marginality within institutional hegemony perpetuate the structural constraints that produce conformity to the status quo. So, how can critical resistance become part of a process for change?

Critical Resistance in Nursing Education

Critical resistance in nursing education is already developing in New Zealand as part of critical pedagogical work in cultural safety. We use classroom strategies to create a "discourse of possibility," such as small tutorial groups with the same nurse educator, debate and critique of issues that relate to domination and oppression as they arise from everyday experiences and the media, reflective journaling that serves as an account of one's historical journey in cultural safety, and presentation of ideas for cultural assessment in various formats (for example, through video, poetry, stories, drawings, booklets, and drama). Nurse educators could also form narrative groups among themselves, which would create a space for students, teachers and clinicians to come together and share personal narratives about their work of critical resistance. Our experiences need to be both spoken and written about because New Zealand leads the way in addressing cultural safety issues in nursing education.

An example of a narrative approach has already been undertaken by Professor Nancy Diekelmann through her research in Narrative Pedagogy at various pilot sites (Diekelmann, 2001). Another example is the Personal Narratives Group (1989)—a collective of academic women and students that came together at the Center of Advanced Feminist Studies at the University of Minnesota. The group had a commitment to grounding feminist theory in women's lived experiences and considered women's personal narratives as the primary source for feminist research and the interpretation of text.

Narrative groups need to be inclusive, not exclusive, so that many stories can be told. By coming together to create, recreate, and share our life stories we can construct a context for listening, interpreting, and reflecting that does not exist in the work environment. In viewing our work as critical work, nurse educators can see that the resistance of our students and colleagues is important for building an empowering critical resistance. When we explore how our multiple subjectivities as teachers contribute to the oppositional but reciprocal aspects of resistance and accommodation in ourselves and students, we can see and hear the different ways that interlocking oppressions can present conflict and paradox for us. By sharing stories of teaching and learning practices, nurse educators and students are able to locate themselves within their experiences, use their experiences as tools for learning and teaching, validate and affirm their experiences, and provide a transforming experience and means of resisting oppression for themselves and others.

Autobiography and Critical Resistance

I have been able to critically reflect on how my lived experiences of resisting and accommodating oppression in nursing challenge sexist, racist, and classist hegemony. I have endeavored to synthesize theories of oppression, theories of resistance, critical feminist theory, and my autobiographical narrative exemplars using a heuristic research method, while recognizing that my account of resisting and accommodating oppression is "positioned and partial" (Middleton, 1993). This account I have labeled the CRP.

In addition to answering the question how can nurse educators resist oppression, I have developed a CRP, which I suggest provides an alternative vision for a counter-hegemonic education. At the same time, I recognize that as a nurse educator I am positioned within multiple and contradictory power relations. Although this research is a turning point for me, it is only part of an ongoing journey in the development of a CRP in nursing education. Questions remain to be answered, such as: How will nurse educators respond to the idea of a CRP? How can a CRP be implemented internationally in nursing education? How do nurse educators who identify themselves as critical resisters thrive and survive? What are the common practices that nurse educators use in encouraging and sustaining resistance?

Implications for Other Health Professionals

While the focus of this chapter has been on the development of a CRP in nursing education, the markers comprising this pathway are relevant to other health professions as well. The CRP is open to interpretation and development by individuals or groups involved in teaching and learning in all health professions. Issues of race, gender, and class are part of our personal and professional environments and critical resistance is not the sole domain of nursing. Health and education institutions are hegemonic structures that maintain the ideas, values, and beliefs of dominant groups in society, ideas, values, and beliefs that are embedded in the consciousness of the people who work in them. The questions outlined in the previous section might also be posed for all health professionals. How might they respond to the notion of a CRP? Do they identify themselves as critical resisters in healthcare and education? Could it be implemented as part of their education programs? As members of a multidisciplinary team in health practice, it is imperative that we work together to critique the discourses of dominance (e.g., power, colonization) that influence the health and illness (and education) outcomes of consumers (patients, students). This critique could take the form of working more effectively with issues of difference, rather than trying to marginalize or resist them. Opie (1999) also suggests that this process can work toward flattening professional hierarchies.

Conclusion

This study has assisted me in critiquing the hegemonic structures in my society, and in reflecting on strategies for critical resistance in nursing education. As nurse educators, we need to overcome the contradictory paradoxical nature of our job and develop strategies that address issues of tension between social structures and agency, as well as our individual resistances to, or accommodation of, oppression. Nursing education has been handicapped for too long by an oppressive model that is based on control, conformity, and resistance. A CRP offers us an opportunity to free ourselves of the idea that we are "masters of truth and justice and [move] more toward creating a space where those directly involved can act and speak on their own behalf" (Lather, 1991, p. 164).

This chapter will, I hope, be useful for all health professionals by drawing attention to the contradictions, conflicts, and tensions of multiple oppressions that are present in our lives. I also hope that it may inspire others to recognize that we are active agents capable of addressing multiple oppressions through a CRP. However, in no way is this pathway to be considered canonical—that is, the only way to resist oppression. I suggest that it be left open to different and multiple interpretations.

I intend to continue this research by examining other positions and interpretations of a CRP. I wish to explore the emerging markers and develop the pathway further by talking with other nurse educators about their lived experiences as critical resisters. My current research explores the life stories of six nurse educators who teach for social change in New Zealand. Using collaborative theorizing, we will build on existing knowledges to create new nursing knowledge (Diekelmann, 2001; Lather, 1991; Middleton, 1993). We will also make visible the interlocking oppressions that separate us, but at the same time unite us— as women, as nurses, and as educators.

Notes

1. Cultural safety was introduced into undergraduate nursing curricula by the Nursing Council of New Zealand in 1992. It focuses on addressing issues of personal and institutional power, and acknowledging and respecting difference in patients/clients to ensure that our practice does not demean, diminish, or disempower them.

2. Maori is the collective name for the indigenous people of New Zealand.

3. Ward sister was a term used until the 1970s when it changed to charge nurse or nurse manager of a unit.

4. Matron was the head nurse of a hospital.

5. The Health and Disability Act provides consumers with an advocacy and complaint process.

6. Pakeha is a term conscientized Europeans call themselves rather than "North American/European." Originally coined by Maori, it refers to the tall, white sails of the early sailing ships that brought the first white settlers to New Zealand.

7. Rugby football has been the most popular male sport in New Zealand since the early days of white settlement.

8. The Nursing Council of New Zealand is a regulatory and statutory body that registers nurses, and approves and audits nursing curricula.

9. The personal grievance case was still before the Employment Court.

10. The Treaty of Waitangi was signed in 1840 by the British Crown and Maori leaders. It legalized European settlement and is regarded by many as the founding document of Aoteaora/New Zealand.

References

Abrums, M., & Leppa, C. (2001). Beyond cultural competence: Teaching about race, gender, class, and sexual orientation. *Journal of Nursing Education, 40*(6), 270–275.

Apple, M. (1993). *Official knowledge: Democratic education in a conservative age.* New York: Routledge.

Arnot, M., & Weiler, K. (Eds.). (1993). *Feminism and social justice in education: international perspectives.* London: Falmer.

Baisnée, V. (1997). *Gendered resistance. The autobiographies of Simone de Beauvoir, Maya Angelou, Janet Frame and Marguerite Duras.* Amsterdam: Rodopi.

Baker, C., & Diekelmann, N. (1994). Connecting conversations of caring: Recalling the narrative to clinical practice. *Nursing Outlook, 42*(2), 65–70.

Banks-Wallace, J. (1998). Emancipatory potential of storytelling in a group. *Image: Journal of Nursing Scholarship, 30*(1), 17–21.

Battersby, D., & Hemmings, L. (1990). Oppression, contestation and resistance in nursing: A case study. Paper presented at the University of Waikato, Hamilton, New Zealand.

Belenky, M., Clinchy, B., Goldberger, N., & Tarule, J. (1986). *Women's ways of knowing.* New York: Basic Books.

Benner, P. (1984). *From novice to expert: Excellence and power in clinical nursing practice.* Menlo Park, CA: Addison-Wesley.

Bent, K. (1993). Perspectives on critical and feminist theory in developing nursing praxis. *Journal of Professional Nursing, 9*(5), 296–303.

Berlak, A. (1989). Teaching for outrage and empathy in the liberal arts. *Educational Foundations, 3*(1), 69–93.

Bevis, E., & Watson, J. (1989). *Toward a caring curriculum: A new pedagogy for nursing.* New York: National League for Nursing Press.

Boler, M. (1999). Posing feminist queries to Freire. In P. Roberts. (Ed.), *Paulo Freire, Politics and Pedagogy: Reflections from Aotearoa-New Zealand.* Palmerston North, New Zealand: Dunmore.

Boutain, D. (1999). Critical nursing scholarship: Exploring critical social theory with African American studies. *Advances in Nursing Science, 21*(4), 37–47.

Brettell, C. (1997). Blurred genres and blended voices: Life history, biography, autobiography, and the auto/ethnography of women's lives. In D. Reed-Danahy (Ed.), *Auto/ethnography: Rewriting the self and the social.* Oxford: Berg.

Bunkle, P. (1992). Becoming knowers: Feminism, science and medicine. In R. du Plessis (Ed.), *Feminist Voices: Women's studies texts for Aotearoa-New Zealand.* Auckland, New Zealand: Oxford University Press.

Buresh, B., & Gordon, S. (2000). *From silence to voice: What nurses know and must communicate to the public.* Ottawa: Canadian Nurses Association.

Chesler, P. (1989). *Women and madness* (2nd ed.). New York: Harcourt Brace Jovanovich.

Church, K. (1995). *Forbidden narratives: Critical autobiography as social science.* Luxembourg: Gordon & Breach.

Clandinin, J., & Connelly, M. (1998). Personal experience methods. In N. Denzin & Y. Lincoln (Eds.), *Collecting and interpreting qualitative materials.* Thousand Oaks, CA: Sage.

Clandinin, J., & Connelly, M. (2000). *Narrative inquiry: Experience and story in qualitative research.* San Francisco: Jossey Bass.

Clare, J. (1991). *Teaching and learning in nursing education: A critical approach.* Unpublished doctoral thesis, Massey University, Palmerston North, New Zealand.

Cleary, D. (2001). Oppression, power, inequality: An interdisciplinary approach. *Teaching Sociology, 29*(1), 36–47.

Clements, P. (1999). Autobiographical research and the emergence of the fictive voice. *Cambridge Journal of Education, 29*(1), 21–32.

Cortazzi, M. (1993). *Narrative analysis.* London: Falmer.

David, B. (2000). Nursing's gender politics: Reformulating the footnotes. *Advances in Nursing Science, 23*(1), 83–93.

Denzin, N. (1989). *Interpretive biography.* Newbury Park, CA: Sage.

Denzin, N., & Lincoln,Y. (Eds.). (1998). *Collecting and interpreting qualitative materials.* Thousand Oaks, CA: Sage.

Derman-Sparks, L., & Phillips, C. (1997). *Teaching/learning anti-racism: A developmental approach.* New York: Teachers College Press.

Diekelmann, N. (1993). Behavioral pedagogy: Heideggerian hermeneutical analysis of the lived experiences of students and teachers in baccalaureate nursing education. *Journal of Nursing Education, 32*(6), 245–250.

Diekelmann, N. (1995). Reawakening thinking: Is traditional pedagogy nearing completion? *Journal of Nursing Education, 34*(5), 195–196.

Diekelmann, N. (2001). Narrative pedagogy: Heideggerian hermeneutical analyses of the lived experiences of students, teachers and clinicians. *Advances in Nursing Science, 23*(3), 53–71.

Diekelmann, N., & Diekelmann, J. (forthcoming). *Schooling learning teaching: Toward a Narrative Pedagogy.* Madison: University of Wisconsin Press.

Duffy, E. (1995). Horizontal violence: A conundrum for nursing. *Collegian, 2*(2), 5-17.

Elliott, E. (1989). The discourse of nursing: A case of silencing. *Nursing and Health Care, 10*(4), 539–543.

Ellis, C., & Flaherty, M. (Eds.). (1992). *Investigating subjectivity: Research on lived experience.* Newbury Park, CA: Sage.

Ellsworth, E. (1989). Why doesn't this feel empowering? Working through the repressive myths of critical pedagogy. *Harvard Educational Review, 59*(3), 297–324.

Ellsworth, E. (1997). *Teaching positions: Difference, pedagogy, and the power of address.* New York: Teachers College Press.

Emden, C. (1998). Theoretical perspectives on narrative inquiry. *Collegian, 5*(2), 30–35.

Estés, C. (1992). *Women who run with the wolves: Myths and stories of the wild woman archetype.* London: Rider.

Fletcher, S. (2000). *Education and emancipation: Theory and practice in a new constellation.* New York: Teachers College Press.

Foucault, M. (1977). The political function of the intellectual. *Radical Philosophy, 17,* 12–14.

Fox, R. (1994). *Cultural safety: Speaking the unspeakable. A monograph of one person's reality.* Unpublished paper.

Freire, P. (1972). *Pedagogy of the oppressed.* (M. B. Ramos, Trans.). Harmondsworth, UK: Penguin.

Freire, P. (1973). *Education for critical consciousness.* New York: Seabury.

Frid, I., Ohlen, J., & Bergbom, I. (2000). On the use of narratives in nursing research. *Journal of Advanced Nursing, 32*(3), 695–703.

Gewirtz, D. (1991). Analyses of racism and sexism in education and strategies for change. *British Journal of Sociology of Education, 12*(2), 183–201.

Giroux, H. (1983). Theories of reproduction and resistance in the new sociology of education: A critical analysis. *Harvard Educational Review, 53*(3), 257–293.

Glass, N. (1994). *Breaking a social silence, women's emerging and disruptive voices: A feminist critique of post-registration nursing education in rural Australia.* Unpublished doctoral thesis, University of New South Wales, Australia.

Glass, N. (1997). Horizontal violence in nursing: Celebrating conscious healing strategies. *Australian Journal of Holistic Nursing, 4*(2), 15–23.

Glass, N. (1998). Becoming de-silenced and reclaiming voice: Women nurses speak out. In H. Keleher & F. McInerney (Eds), *Nursing Matters: Critical Sociological Perspectives.* Melbourne: Churchill Livingstone.

Gore, J. (1993). *The struggle for pedagogies: Critical and feminist discourse as regimes of truth.* New York: Routledge.

Gramsci, A. (1971). *Selections from the prison notebooks.* (Q. Hoare & G. Smith, Eds. & Trans.). New York: International Publishers.

Greene, M. (1988). *The dialectic of freedom.* New York: Teachers College Press.

Guba, E., & Lincoln, Y. (1989). *Fourth generation evaluation.* Newbury Park, CA: Sage.

Hall, J., Stevens, P., & Meleis, A. (1994). Marginalization: A guiding concept for valuing diversity in nursing knowledge development. *Advances in Nursing Science, 16*(4), 23–41.

Harden, J. (1996). Enlightenment, empowerment and emancipation: The case for critical pedagogy in nursing education. *Nurse Education Today, 16*(1), 32–37.

Hatch, J., & Wisniewski, R. (Eds.). (1995). *Life history and narrative.* London: Falmer.

hooks, b. (1984). *From margin to center.* Boston: South End.

hooks, b. (1995). *Killing rage: Ending racism.* New York: Henry Holt.

hooks, b. (2000). *Where we stand: Class matters.* New York: Routledge.

Hutchinson, S. (1990). Responsible subversion: A study of rule bending among nurses. *Scholarly Inquiry for Nursing Practice, 4*(1), 3–22.

Ironside, P. (2001). Creating a research base for nursing education: An interpretive review of conventional, critical, feminist, postmodern, and phenomenological practices. *Advances in Nursing Science, 23*(3), 72–87.

Johnstone, M.-J. (1999). Reflective topical autobiography: An under utilized interpretive research method in nursing, *Collegian, 6*(1), 24–29.

Jones, A. (1991). *"At school I've got a chance": Culture/privilege: Pacific Islands and Pakeha girls at school.* Palmerston North, New Zealand: Dunmore Press.

Keddy, B. (1995). Feminist teaching and the older nurse: The journey from resistance through anger to hope. *Journal of Advanced Nursing, 21*(4), 690–694.

Kirton, J. (1997). *Paakeha/Tauiwi: Seeing the "unseen": Critical analysis of links between discourse, identity, "blindness" and encultured racism.* Kirikiriroa, New Zealand: Waikato Antiracism Coalition.

Kleffel, D. (1991). An ecofeminist analysis of nursing knowledge. *Nursing Forum, 26*(4), 5–18.

Koch, T. (1998). Story telling: Is it really research? *Journal of Advanced Nursing, 28*(6), 1182–1190.

Koch, T., & Harrington, A. (1998). Reconceptualising rigor: The case for reflexivity. *Journal of Advanced Nursing, 28*(4), 882–890.

Kuokkanen, L., & Leino-Kilpi, H. (2000). Power and empowerment in nursing: Three theoretical approaches. *Journal of Advanced Nursing, 31*(1), 235–241.

Lather, P. (1991). *Getting smart: Feminist research and pedagogy with/in the postmodern.* New York: Routledge.

Lee, M., & Saeed, I. (2001). Oppression and horizontal violence: The case of nurses in Pakistan. *Nursing Forum, 36*(1), 15–24.

Lewis, M. (1990). Interrupting patriarchy: Politics, resistance and transformation in the feminist classroom. *Harvard Educational Review, 60*(4), 467–488.

Lewis, M., & Simon, R. (1986). A discourse not intended for her: Learning and teaching within patriarchy. *Harvard Educational Review, 56*(4), 457–472.

Luke, C., & Gore, J. (Eds.). (1992). *Feminisms and critical pedagogy.* New York: Routledge.

McEldowney, R. (1992). *A new lamp is shining: Life histories of five feminist nurse educators.* Unpublished paper.

McFadden, M. (1995). Resistance to schooling and educational outcomes—questions of structure and agency. *British Journal of Sociology of Education, 16*(3), 293–308.

McRobbie, A. (1978). Working class girls and the culture of femininity. In Women's Studies Group (Eds.), *Women take issue: Aspects of women's subordination.* London: Hutchinson.

Middleton, S. (1993). *Educating feminists: Life histories and pedagogy.* New York: Teachers College Press.

Moustakas, C. (1990). *Heuristic research: Design, methods and application.* Newbury Park, CA: Sage.

Munns, G., & McFadden, M. (2000). First chance, second chance or last chance? Resistance and response to education. *British Journal of Sociology of Education, 21*(1), 59–75.

Munro, P. (1998). *Subject to fiction: Women teachers' life history narratives and the cultural politics of resistance.* Buckingham, UK: Open University Press.

Ng, R., Staton, P., & Scane, J. (Eds.). (1995). *Antiracism, feminism, and critical approaches to education.* Westport, CT: Bergin & Garvey.

Nicholson, L. (1990). (Ed.). *Feminism/postmodernism.* New York: Routledge.

Opie, A. (1999). Knowledge-based teamwork. In P. Davis & K. Dew (Eds.), *Health and Society in Aotearoa New Zealand* (pp. 181–198). Auckland, New Zealand: Oxford University Press.

Parker, J., & Gardner, G. (1992). The silence and the silencing of the nurse's voice: A reading of patient progress notes. *The Australian Journal of Advanced Nursing, 9*(2), 3–9.

Pelissier, C. (1992). *Accommodation and resistance among recipients and workers: An ethnographic analysis of women and welfare.* Unpublished doctoral dissertation, Michigan State University, East Lansing.

Popkewitz, T., & Fendler, L. (1999). *Critical theories in education: Changing terrains of knowledge and politics.* New York: Routledge.

Ramsden, I. (1992). *Kawa Whakaruruhau. Guidelines for nursing and midwifery education.* Wellington: Nursing Council of New Zealand.

Rather, M. (1994). "Schooling for oppression": A critical hermeneutic analysis of the lived experience of the returning RN student. *Journal of Nursing Education, 33*(6), 263–271.

Reason, P. (Ed.). (1988). *Human inquiry in action: Developments in new paradigm research.* London: Sage.

Ribbens, J. (1993). Facts or fictions? Aspects of the use of autobiographical writing in undergraduate sociology. *Sociology, 27*(1), 81–92.

Rich, A. (1979). *On lies, secrets, and silence: Selected prose, 1966–1978.* New York: W. W. Norton.

Richardson, L. (1998). Writing. A method of inquiry. In N. Denzin and Y. Lincoln (Eds.), *Collecting and interpreting qualitative materials.* Thousand Oaks, CA: Sage.

Roberts, S. (1983). Oppressed group behaviour: Implications for nursing. *Advances in Nursing Science, 5*(4), 21–30.

Roberts, S. (1997). Nurse executives in the 1990s: Empowered or oppressed? *Nursing Administration Quarterly, 22*(1), 64–71.

Roberts, S. (2000). Development of a positive professional identity: Liberating oneself from the oppressor within. *Advances in Nursing Science, 22*(4), 71–82.

Ruffing-Rahal, M. (1992). Incorporating feminism into the graduate curriculum. *Journal of Nursing Education, 31*(6), 247–252.

Sandelowski, M. (1991). Telling stories: Narrative approaches in qualitative research. *Image: Journal of Nursing Scholarship, 23*(3), 161–166.

Scarry, K. (1999). Nursing elective: Balancing caregiving in oppressive systems. *Journal of Nursing Education, 38*(9), 423–427.

Skillings, L. (1992). Perceptions and feelings of nurses about horizontal violence as an expression of oppressed group behaviour. In J. Thompson, D. Allen, & L. Rodriguez-Fisher (Eds.), *Critique, resistance and action: Working papers in the politics of nursing*. New York: National League for Nursing.

Smith, L. (1993). Getting out from down under: Maori women, education and the struggles for Mana Wahine. In M. Arnot & K. Weiler (Eds.), *Feminism and social justice in education: International perspectives*. London: Falmer Press.

Starhawk. (1987). *Truth or dare: Encounters with power, authority, and mystery*. San Francisco: Harper & Row.

Starhawk. (1990). *Dreaming the dark: Magic, sex, and politics*. London: Unwin Hyman.

Steen, M. (1991). Historical perspectives on women and mental illness and prevention of depression in women, using a feminist framework. *Issues in Mental Health Nursing, 12*(4), 359–374.

Tatum, B. (1992). Talking about race, learning about racism: The application of racial identity development in the classroom. *Harvard Educational Review, 62*(1), 1–24.

Titus, J. (2000). Engaging student resistance to feminism: "How is this stuff going to make us better teachers?" *Gender and Education, 12*(1), 21–37.

Varcoe, C. (1996). Theorizing oppression: Implications for nursing research on violence against women. *Canadian Journal of Nursing Research, 28*(1), 61–78.

Warnke, G. (1993). Feminism and hermeneutics. *Hypatia, 8*(1), 81–97.

Watson, J. (1990). The moral failure of the patriarchy. *Nursing Outlook, 38*(2), 62–66.

Weiler, K. (1988). *Women teaching for change: Gender, class, and power*. South Hadley, MA: Bergin & Garvey.

Weiler, K. (1993). Feminism and the struggle for a democratic education: A view from the United States. In M. Arnot, & K. Weiler (Eds.), *Feminism and social justice in education: International perspectives*. London: Falmer Press.

White, K. (1999). Theories about health and society. In P. Davis & K. Dew. (Eds.), *Health and Society in Aotearoa New Zealand*. Auckland, New Zealand: Oxford University Press.

Willis, P. (1977). *Learning to labour: How working class lads get working class jobs*. Farnborough, U. K.: Saxon House.

Yeatman, A. (1993). Voice and representation in the politics of difference. In S. Gunew, & A. Yeatman (Eds.), *Feminism and the politics of difference*. Wellington, New Zealand: Bridget Williams.

Young, I. (1990). *Justice and the politics of difference*. Princeton, NJ: Princeton University Press.

5

Teaching as Nourishment for Complex Thought

Approaches for Classroom and Practice Built on Postformal Theory and the Creation of Community

Jan D. Sinnott

"Once Upon a Time . . . ," or How I Learned to Teach More Effectively, Honoring Mind *and* Heart

My (Mis-)Adventures as a Traditional College Professor

When I was nearing the end of my Ph.D. program in Life Span Developmental Psychology, I did not think of teaching as "nourishment for life." But I did think teaching was good for passing information on from the informed to the uninformed. This was how I had always experienced it.

One day I had what I thought was a bright idea: I decided to create a course that our department did not yet offer, a course in my area of interest: psychology of aging. I talked up the idea to a fellow graduate student with similar interests. We were both interested but a little hesitant. We had acted as teaching assistants before, but that was very different from creating and teaching a new course by ourselves. I also should mention that this adventure occurred in that time long, long ago when there were no textbooks on the "Psychology of Aging." This meant that we personally had to compile all meaningful material and summarize it in some reasonable way before we presented it to students.

232

The idea was approved; the new course could begin. But, although getting the approval took considerable effort, the task of preparing for the class took even more. Being diligent, compulsive graduate students had paid off in our careers so far, so my colleague and I continued on that path. Articles and books and Xerox copies began to take over my house. And, having found all this information, we seem to have unconsciously sworn to use every bit of it! We would be thorough! We would present students with the whole picture of what was known about the psychology of aging!

I apologize to those of you readers with any classroom teaching experience. I'm sure your anxiety is already beginning to mount. You know what is coming when professors, especially young and inexperienced ones, start to think like this, and it is not good for learning.

The first day of class finally came, and it led to the first week and then the first month. Each class day I or my colleague would arrive with reams of notes and articles, and lecture, lecture, lecture. Rapidly! No bit of information would be ignored! Students wrote until their hands cramped and the board was full. But we lecturers felt great! We were doing a great job!

The discussion of "death and dying" came near the end of the course, naturally. I gave my usual jam-packed lecture and the sound of note-taking instruments was intense. But toward the end of the class something very unusual happened, something that ultimately caused me to abandon my extensive notes: an extremely capable student burst into tears and said she had to drop the class. As she ran from the room I asked her to please meet me after class so we could talk. I was shocked. She did wait, and after class I talked with her further.

Unknown to me, during the current semester this student had been the main caretaker of an older ailing relative who had just died in the last few days. She had not said anything about this significant experience when we'd lectured on caretaking or on cognitive and physical changes. But, upon reflection, I realized that, after all, how could she say anything? We lecturers had never stopped talking! Now she was pouring out the whole story of the relative's dying process and her experience of it. I knew what she was talking about. I had also been through some similar events, and we could relate to each other on that basis. But the thing that impressed me the most (in my role as a professor) was the richness she brought to the material we were discussing that day in class.

The studies had been interesting, but her real-life story was much more interesting. It made the conflicted feelings and the confusions generated by the real event of a death come to life in a way that a study report could not. "I just wish I could tell people what it's really like," she said. And I knew she was right, for many reasons. I asked her if she wanted that chance to "tell people what it's really like," and she said yes, she very much did.

The next class, as usual, students came in ready to hear a lecture and to take voluminous notes. Some of them had that distracted, abstract look on their faces, the look that said that the real world of life and emotions and relationships was far, far away from this room. But they were in for a surprise. We would not "cover" quite as many studies today. They found that the desks were now in a circle, not in rows, since I had wanted the presenting student to feel less conspicuous than she might if she stood in the front of the room. So sitting at one of them was my student who was about to tell her story. We were going to have an unforgettable discussion, and many students were going to feel more like whole human beings.

In the end students agreed that this was a class in which they really learned a lot. They synthesized material and analyzed research and theory critically as they considered the very real "case" of their fellow student and her dying relative. And, from later reports, some of these students were going to remember this material better than any other material from their college careers. Teaching was becoming "nourishment for life."

This was my first realization that "wasting time" not lecturing could be very useful for students and could open up new avenues of learning. Brainwashed as I was by my formal education, I had never considered the educational value of a personal story. That day I began to question what brings about learning. The experience created new challenges, of course, such as how to answer those ever popular "will this be on the final exam?" questions. I can't say I always faced the challenges well; for example, I just used my prepared multiple choice questions for the final exam in that course on aging I just described. But overall this was the beginning of a new part of my learning process as a professor. I was beginning to question my methods and to see that a more complex style than simply lecturing was needed if student learning was to be maximized. I had no theoretical underpinning for that new style yet, and I did not have lots of methods, but as it turned out I was on a better—though riskier—track.

Taking Chances

Even if it proves ultimately more beneficial than sticking with traditional lectures, changing to a professorial teaching style that incorporates something different and "more human" is risky business. Students who know how to "perform" to get that "A" are distressed because the rules seem to have changed. Student ratings might be at risk. More traditional fellow faculty, observing classes for tenure-related purposes, might be confused. (After all, all that noise accompanying activities such as lively student discussions might sound like chaos or a group out of control.) Exams might be harder to create.

I found that deviating from the "norm" in teaching college classes was risky business in many ways, especially at that particular time in the evolution of higher education teaching practices. Those of you who have been on a tenure track, hoping for tenure some day, might remember how carefully you began to act as you got closer to your goal. If that committee did not approve of what you were doing in class, all your innovations wouldn't be of help to any future students because you would be gone! (As you might guess, philosophically I tend to side with those who believe that the struggle for tenure limits academic freedom on the grounds that academics are inclined to become conservative due to fear that tenure will not be attained. Some would argue that by the time an academic secures tenure, he or she has forgotten how to be innovative and has become very conservative!)

Changes in my own courses evolved slowly since not all of those new ideas worked out well and they were not necessarily welcomed. Still, changes in my teaching methods did continue little by little, in the direction of actively engaging the whole mind and heart and spirit and social beings of students in college.

The following section will provide you with a theoretical basis for such experimentation. As it happened, my cognitive developmental research in the evolution of complex "wise" thought overlapped, to some extent, with the teaching methods I was devising for class. The yearning for community, which many of us feel in today's vast global society, is something students experience, too, and the methods I learned to draw on make use of communities of learners. This search for community will be described as it relates to teaching and learning. I'll share with you some methods, and some stories of student responses to them. I'll tie these thoughts and descriptions to the field of healthcare in two ways: by discussing the training of healthcare providers and how healthcare providers teach clients and patients.

First Main Point: My Theory Directs My Teaching Style

There are theoretical underpinnings for the idea of teaching as nourishment for complex thought. As I studied the development of complex thought in adulthood, which is my main research focus, I developed my Theory of Postformal Thought (see Sinnott, 1998b, for a summary of the first 20 years' thinking and research, as well as for applications; see the bibliography for other references). This theory, in turn, is consistent with the world views of the new science models. These world views are informed by a more complex and useful understanding of the learner–teacher relationship than that which is the basis for lecture methods. The Theory of Postformal Thought describes what happens cognitively as adults learn to think and adaptively function, and as they learn to use the scientific logic of the new physics world, as opposed to that confined to the Newtonian physics "local reality," in real life.

Postformal Thought is key to adult development, learning, and wisdom. It is based on an understanding of reality like that which permeates modern sciences. The concepts and skills of Postformal Thought derive from cognitive-developmental theory, native wisdom traditions, "new" sciences such as quantum physics, chaos theory, theories of self-organizing systems, and general systems theory. I believe that teaching adults to think postformally should be an important basic goal whenever we teach them in the university setting or in any other contexts because it allows us to teach the whole human.

Furthermore, I believe that the cognitive skill set that accompanies thinking postformally is the basis of many of the new approaches to education and the new theories of intelligence. Postformal thinking operations (or skills) also are models of the thinking skills necessary to understand modern scientific approaches such as quantum physics, general systems theory, chaos theory, and theories of self-regulating systems (see For Further Reading for selected references). Postformal thinking skills are needed to allow us to be humanistic, honoring the whole multi-faceted person in our educational endeavors.

To summarize the argument I am about to make here, Postformal Thought describes certain cognitive operations. These operations constitute the means for knowing (in the humanistic, holistic sense) complex realities like those of modern sciences such as quantum physics, as well as those of the emotions and human relations. These operations are similar to the underpinnings of some new views of education. This useful way of thinking can be fostered by educational systems to enhance students' abilities to function as developing human beings in the postmodern world.

Over a period of 25 years of study I created the theory of complex Postformal Thought as a way of describing several specific phenomena that would cognitively model the step beyond "formal operational logic" (developed in adolescence) and describe the thinking of mature adult thinkers. I wanted to cognitively model the wise thinking possessed by at least some of my older relatives, friends, and research respondents. I wanted to cognitively model certain logical aspects of the thinking of great twentieth century scientists such as Albert Einstein. And I wanted to cognitively model some logical aspects of intense, even intimate, long-term interpersonal interactions that were successful. As a university professor I also saw that I could help students acquire these postformal skills and that those who had such skills were more successful in their intellectual and interpersonal pursuits. The whole thrust of this research and scholarship was to capture the thinking and teaching related to positive outcomes, and I feel confident that the concept of Postformal Thought is related to, and important to, these significant positive outcomes and should be taught.

Definition and Description of Postformal Thought

Postformal complex thought and the research underlying it are described in my 1998 book, *The Development of Logic in Adulthood: Postformal Thought and Its Applications*. The book outlines the entire Theory of Postformal Thought. Some references that explain this work further are as follows: Sinnott, 1981, 1984, 1989, 1990, 1991a, 1991b, 1993a, 1993b, 1994a, 1994b, 1996, 1997, 1998a, 1998b, 2000, in preparation a, in preparation b; Sinnott & Johnson, 1996a, Sinnott & Johnson,

1996b. These materials also describe the nature of the individual think-ing operations that together make up Postformal Thought.

Postformal Thought is a type of complex logical thinking that devel-ops in adulthood when we interact with other people whose views about some aspect of reality are different from ours. Of course this kind of interaction is what should occur in educational experiences. Postformal Thought builds upon concrete and formal (scientific) Piagetian thought. It allows a person to deal with everyday logical contradictions by en-abling that person to understand that reality and the meaning of events are cocreated. Both objectivity and a necessary subjectivity are useful in our epistemological understanding of the world. Postformal Thought lets an adult bridge two contradictory "scientifically" logical positions and reach an adaptive synthesis of them through a higher-order logic. The adult then goes on to live the larger reality. So the larger reality eventually becomes "true" with the passage of time. Postformal Thought includes a necessary subjectivity, which means that the knower under-stands that "truth" is partially a creation of the one who knows it.

Postformal Thought seems to develop later in life, after a certain amount of intellectual and interpersonal experience. For example, only after experiencing intimate relationships and the shared, mutually con-structed logics about the reality of intimate life together can a person be experienced enough to know that "If I think of you as an untrustworthy partner, then treat you that way, you are likely to truly become an un-trustworthy partner."

Here is another example. When I begin teaching a college class, the class and I begin to structure our relationship. We decide on the nature of our relationship, act on our view of it, and mutually continue to create it in the days that follow. The various views held by class members and by me form several contradictory logical systems about the reality of our relationship in the class. One student may see me as a surrogate parent and act within the formal logic inherent in that vision, to which I might respond by becoming more and more parental. Another student may logically construct me as a buddy and act within that logical system, to which I might respond by being a buddy too, or by being even more parental to compensate. I might view the class as stimulating or not, and teach in such a way as to make them either! The result over the course of a semester will be a truth about the nature of my relationship with this class that is cocreated by the class and me.

While postformal complex thought is stimulated by interpersona interactions among thinkers, once it becomes a thinking tool for a person it may be applied to any kind of knowing situation, not just interpersonal ones. I may learn to use the tool of complex Postformal Thought through interactions with my spouse and go on to use it to think about Newtonian versus quantum physics. Just as the tool of scientific logic can be used in any context, so too the tool of complex Postformal Thought can be used in any context. Of course, decisions need to be made about whether it is an appropriate tool in a given context. Complex Postformal Thought that orders several contradictory logical systems is probably unnecessary for less epistemologically demanding tasks such as rote memorization of an agreed-upon body of material.

Nine thinking operations make up Postformal Thought. Rationale for inclusion of these operations is given in my summary book about the theory (Sinnott, 1998b). The operations include: *metatheory shift, problem definition, process/product shift, parameter setting, multiple solutions, pragmatism, multiple causality, multiple methods,* and *para-dox.* You can go to the references above to read more about the meaning of each operation, the ways these operations have been tested, and the research that provides an underpinning for these assertions. I will briefly describe each operation here, giving a simple example of each. Notice that the operations will relate to one another, but will simultaneously describe different aspects of the complex thinking process. Notice too that all the operations relate to problem solving, in the broadest sense.

Metatheory shift is the ability to view reality from more than one logical perspective (for example, from both an abstract and a practical perspective, or from a phenomenological and an experimental perspective) when thinking about it. For example, do I think of getting through college as a chance to open my mind to new areas of knowledge, or as collecting 125 credits, or as (of necessity) both?

Problem definition is the realization that there is always more than one way to define a problem since we all see things like problems through our own unique lenses, and that one must define a problem to solve it. For example, I decide as a student that my problem is "how to guess what my professor is putting on the test," or is "how to memorize the names of the researchers in my textbook." Defining the problem in different ways leads to different ways to solve it.

Process/product shift is realizing that I can reach a "content-related" solution to a given problem, and/or a solution that gives me a heuristic or a process that solves many such problems. For example, do I learn the answers for a given exam, or do I learn a set of general study skills, or both?

Parameter setting is the realization that one must choose aspects of the problem context to be considered or ignored in finding a solution. For example, I decide to limit my study for a test to two hours, looking at the material in chapter 3, going easy on the research methods section but memorizing all the researchers' names and all the terms. I also ask the question, "How am I deciding to approach exams this way? Is there a better way?" All these decisions and questions set limits for my study (that is, for my solution to the problem).

Multiple solutions means that I can generate several solutions, based on several ways of viewing the problem. For example, I can solve the problem of when to study for an exam in three ways: study the night before, at 8:00 P.M.; study during the morning of the test, at 4:00 A.M.; or study gradually over several days.

Pragmatism in this case means that I am able to evaluate the solutions that I create for the problem, and then select one that is "best" by some definition. For example, once I have solved the problem of when to study for the exam, I am then able, by some criterion, to pick the one that is "best."

Multiple causality is the realization that an event can be the result of several causes. For example, when I receive a low grade on a exam, I can consider whether the D is due to sleep deprivation, poor teaching, limited ability, confusion about the chapters on the test, or all of the above.

Multiple methods is the realization that there are several means to the same solution of a problem. For example, I can do better on the next exam by studying longer, by getting more sleep, or by cheating.

Paradox is realizing that contradictions are inherent in reality, and realizing that the broader view of an event can eliminate them. For example, I see that if I stay on the gymnastics team I can keep my scholarship and stay in college, but then I might fail more subjects and might need to leave college (due to lack of study time because I would be attending all those team practices). In this situation I can only resolve my dilemma by reasoning about it at a more complex level, perhaps setting a new goal by asking "What will give me the most satisfying life, and how do I get there?"

The development of Postformal Thought helps explain how college students change their thinking styles as they go through the university experience. Successful students (for example, see Perry, 1975) are first concrete thinkers who need to know the "right" answers. They want to know the "right" personality theory and the "right" major for them to study. They expect an authority to tell them the answer. Professors become the authority figures who provide answers. Then, second, they become relativistic thinkers, shaken by the apparent disappearance of "Truth" ("no right or wrong answers exist," "no way to decide about Truth," "whatever"). Now they see debates as going on forever, without closure. It doesn't matter which philosophy one professes or which major one takes; it's all the same endless, ongoing debate. Finally, third, they move on to complex thinking, a type of thinking in which they see that a necessary subjectivity is part of decisions about truth. A passionate commitment to the choice of a "reality" leads to making it "real" in the objective world. That complex thinking appears to be Postformal Thought. At that stage they can say "It's up to me to pick 'the right major,' then make a commitment to it, act as if it is the right choice for me, and see if it works out. It does matter what I pick . . . not all majors would suit me. But no authority can tell me which will turn out to be 'right.' In fact, no major will be 'right' unless I commit to it as if some absolute authority told me it is the true major for me!"

This complex kind of thinking skill, once attained in a given context, can be transferred from context to context. The student may have gained insight into the complexity of epistemological truth in the context of choice of a major, or relationships with peers, or as part of student government. However it is gained, the postformal complex thinker is able to use that set of complex thinking skills in all subject areas and contexts, if he or she chooses to apply it to them.

The main characteristics of postformal cognitive operations (Sinnott, 1998b) are: (a) self reference, and (b) the ordering of formal operations. Self-reference is a general term for describing ideas associated with new physics (Wolf, 1981) and alluded to by Hofstadter (1979) using the terms "self-referential games," "jumping out of the system," and "strange loops." The essential notion of self-reference is that we can never completely transcend the built-in limits of our system of knowing and that we come to know that this very fact is true. This means that we somewhat routinely can take into account, in our decisions about truth, the fact that all knowledge has a subjective component and therefore is, of necessity, incomplete. So, any logic we use is a self-referential logic. Yet we must act in spite of being trapped in partial subjectivity. We make a decision about the rules of the game (the nature of truth), then act based on those rules. Once we come to realize what we are doing, we then can consciously use such self-referential thought.

The second characteristic of postformal operations is the ordering of Piagetian formal operations (Inhelder & Piaget, 1958). The higher level postformal system of self-referential truth decisions gives order to lower level formal truth and logic systems. One of these logic systems is somewhat subjectively chosen and imposed on data as "true." For example, Perry (1975) describes advanced college students as "deciding" a certain ethical system is "true," while knowing full well that there is no absolute way of deciding the truth of an ethical system.

In the following example, we might also see a relativistic, self-referential organization of several formal operations systems. An attorney is trying to decide whether to defend a very young child accused of sexually assaulting another child. There is no conclusive physical evidence and no witnesses were present. Both children are adamant in their stories and both have been known to distort the truth to some degree when they were angry with each other. The attorney must make a commitment to a course of action and follow through on it as if that logical system were true. The attorney knows that, when she acts, that logical system may become true due to her actions, and will then become legal "truth" in court as well as an emotional truth for her and the others involved. Formal operations presume logical consistency within a single logical system. Within that single system the implications of the system are absolute. Postformal operations presume somewhat necessarily subjective selection among logically contradictory formal operational systems each of which is internally consistent and absolute

As is true for other Piagetian thinking operations systems, a knower who is capable of using Postformal Thought skips in and out of that type of thinking. Postformal Thought is not always the best way to process a certain experience; it may be that sensorimotor thought (or some other stage of thought) is most adaptive on a given day. Or perhaps a thinker with higher-order thinking skills is being confronted with a new situation for which he or she has no thinking structures to abstract from and no logical systems to choose among, not even sensorimotor logic.

For example, a grandparent of mine had never learned to drive, even though she was a very intelligent woman. When presented with the chance to learn to drive, the first thing she did was to read about it, trying to use formal thought. Although she knew, after her reading, about "defensive driving" and other concepts like the logic of the auto-motive engine, this "higher level" knowledge did not help much when she first tried to engage the clutch and drive away smoothly. In fact, this particular grandmother was so shocked by her first-time, terrible, actual (physical) driving performance, compared to her excellent book understanding, that she panicked and let the car roll out of control until it came to a stop against a huge rock. Learning the sensorimotor skill of getting that stick-shift car out on the road was "lower-level" thinking, but it was the most adaptive kind of thinking for that situation. Using the right level of thought for the occasion may be one thing that people learn as they become postformal.

What characterizes the adaptive power of Postformal Thought? Why is it helpful to an adult? How must an adult structure thinking, over and above the operations of formal-operational adolescents, to be in touch with reality and survive? What is important here is not coming to know specific facts, but rather developing general "higher-level" intel-lectual operations, or processes that the knower can use to make existen-tial sense of life and to make life work in situations that go beyond the limits of lower-level thinking.

One key thing competent mature adults seem to need (based on their statements and on observation and task analyses) is to be able to choose one logical model (in other words, one formal operational struc-ture) of the many possible logical models to impose on a given cognitive or emotional reality so that they can make decisions and get on with life. They also need to know that they are making, necessarily, (partly) subjective decisions about reality when they do this. This can be taught in any educational setting.

Selected Applications to Education

In what ways might we apply all this information about these postfor-mal world views to the activity of education in its formal or informal, institutional or casual, primary or secondary or postsecondary forms? The overall application relates to the context of education. There are five areas: relation to the concept of "learning," the methods and philosophies by which teachers teach, the way master teachers reason, the structure of learning institutions, and the way adult learners learn (or fail to learn). Several books contain material that speaks to the topic of this chapter and that is informed by the Theory of Postformal Thought. The reader might wish to examine Kahaney, Janangelo, and Perry's (1993) work on teacher change (including my own chapter); Sinnott's (1994b) handbook of adult life span learning; Sinnott and Cavanaugh's (1991) work on paradigm bridging, especially chapters by Johnson, Lee, and Tanon; and Sinnott and Johnson's (1996a) book on reinventing the university. These are just a few of the novel attempts to assess and improve the state of education in a historical period in which great flexibility is needed in dealing with major changes in and demands on education systems. In my own publications on the issue of education and learning—publications addressing theory, methods, and the structure of the university itself as a teaching institution (e.g., Sinnott, 1993a, 1994b, in preparation b; Sinnott & Johnson, 1996a)—I have stressed the need for the learning and teaching of the postformal process and engagement with the learner to occur in an existentially meaningful context. Transformational learning, as described by Jack Mezirow (2000), and the evolution of the knowing self, as described by Robert Kegan (1982), are examples of the development of and use of Postformal Thought in learning situations of many sorts.

Second Main Point: The Development of Complex Thought Rests upon Building Community in the Learning Situation

Yearning for Community

If you recall the class situation I described at the very beginning of this chapter you'll notice that when the student with the dying relative told her story to the class, a wonderful thing began to happen. That wonderful thing was that a community was created.

The search for community is part of the human yearning to move toward love. We yearn for loving, accepting connections that will facilitate our development. Because I think it is so important a topic, I am preparing a book exploring this search for community and the implications of community for our development (*Moving Toward Love: The Search for Community in a Global Society*, Sinnott, in preparation a). Who is a part of your "community"? What is community? Do you feel that you "belong," that you can identify with a community?

Many have commented that we in the United States suffer from a widespread lack of community and a lack of connections with others. We feel even more isolated when we hear that we now live in a global society or community. Supposedly we are connected to, or interacting with, more and more people each year. College classes grow larger and larger. "Caring" often means caring for more and more strangers with whom few relationships form (e.g., see Pipher, 1999). If there are so many people with whom I am connected, why don't I feel that more people care about me? Why do I sometimes feel lonely? And, in spite of this feeling of loneliness, why do I sometimes wish that e-mails and phone calls would stop arriving? Why do I sometimes feel that those who do make contact with me are superficial or insincere?

One problem that may underlie our current felt lack of community may be that we often have the logical form of community without having community of the heart and spirit to give that form life. For example, I may recite the names of groups I "belong" to while neither caring "from the heart" about those groups or people, nor feeling that they care about me. Another problem may also get in the way of community: I may say that I know who I am, while feeling conflicted about the aspects of my personality that contradict that identity, aspects that I do not yet acknowledge or accept. This can lead to a rejection of others who remind me of disowned parts of myself. There might also be a third impediment to living community: I may say that we all are one and that I love all humanity, but I don't really see the connection between myself and creation, the earth, all beings. I see no transcendent ties that bind us.

The central idea behind the book in preparation is that human adult development always involves the three overlapping activities mentioned above, which are all related to community and feeling a part of a community. All three activities involve a yearning for, a movement toward, and a sharing of love. First, to develop well, we must create a peaceful "inner community" by doing our psychological homework (e.g., learn to love the owned and disowned, the "good" and "bad" aspects of the self). Second, we must create a community with others (e.g., seek to share love with fellow humans). And third, we must create a community of sorts with the Universe/God/Spirit (e.g., seek accord with Universal Love, God, or some other transcendent to attain a spiritual sense of something larger than our own individual selves that ties us to others). All three are important for development at any age (in age-appropriate ways), especially as we move beyond adolescence into adulthood.

Understanding or consciously participating in this process of creating and sharing community has a cognitive side, as do all human behaviors. In this case, our thinking must come to involve cocreating a shared cognitive reality with others (see "Postformal Thought").

Another difficulty in creating community today is that today we live in a global society of rapidly evolving cultures. Our "signals" might be confusing or misread by others. One key distinction is that between objective communities that exist as social organizations and the subjective feelings of community that we have when our own emotions and sense of identity tell us we "belong." It is easy to be confused as to whether we have the former or the latter type of community. In a global society we might enjoy the richness of belonging on a large, multifaceted scale, but run the risk of never feeling that we belong.

Creating Community in the Classroom

Students come into a college classroom to become part of an instant "community" of learners, but they may not feel part of a community there. Traditionally, courses run for a few weeks and restrict dialogue among students, which gives them little opportunity to connect with other learners. If the setting is one of practitioner/client or /patient, the same holds true. Encounters are short and formal and there is little time for feelings to be shared.

It is surprising to me how few adults (students, clients, patients, or others) have experienced feelings of community with fellow humans in spite of the large numbers of people around them. This is especially evident in a hospital or a nursing home setting where large numbers of people buzz in and out of a patient's room while patients report feeling alone and unknown as individuals ("like I was no more than a number or a piece of meat!").

Many modern individuals have had surprisingly little practice in connecting with others. Also, neither teachers, students, practitioners, nor clients have necessarily done their "inner homework" of learning to accept the disowned parts of the self that they can, then, easily project onto others, disrupting relationships. And while some wise persons can bridge the gap among semistrangers because they are able to feel, as a result of membership in a transcendent whole such as the "Family of Humankind," "God," "All Being," or "Nature," connected to others many of us are not yet able to facilitate community feelings in ourselves and others in that wiser way.

Most students in my first psychology of aging class turned out to be hungry for community. They did not know each other. Listening to abstractions as we lectured did not engage their emotions enough to make them feel part of a community. Telling my stories would have helped them feel connected with me even if the storytelling went in only one direction (from teacher to learner), but at that point in my career I was wary of "overstepping the boundaries and getting personal." Students could not readily talk to each other during class, either.

But an objection might arise: why should a class, or any learners and teachers, be a community? Don't these people have a life outside the classroom? These are valid questions, and important ones today. The answer, after all, to the second question might be "no."

When teaching and learning were situated in the ongoing life of students and teachers, we did not have any need to discuss this sort of community in the context of education. Remember "teaching" as "mentoring," or "apprenticeship"? There the flow of information already was contextualized in a relationship and a community of origin. Today my students have been removed from their original contexts and placed into an artificial one in which all key relationships must be created anew. Health practitioners may notice this same dislocation when they interact with clients while doing patient education. The client in the medical office, nursing home, or hospital has been set adrift from his or her community. No one in the new setting may know his or her strengths, weaknesses, past stories, hopes; and no one professional may have time to discover them. The patient who has lost a sense of identity and connections no longer matters as an adult would like to matter.

The existential story has been lost for many modern individuals. Yet we are essentially a "storied people" who live on the basis of our narratives about our existential meaning. To the extent that I know someone's story and someone knows mine, we can communicate, understand, teach, and learn together. Knowing only that you are a student and I am a teacher offers a very narrow platform on which to build new meanings together! It suggests that the mind is separate from the rest of the self, something that new sciences, ancient wisdom, humanistic/existential psychology, and the Theory of Postformal Thought show to be a false assumption. So although the learning environment should not be a substitute for the rest of a full life, the more it honors the fullness of life the more effective it can be. And for those without full, connected lives, for those whose lives have perhaps been artificially narrowed by the constructs of modern life, the learning environment community can be especially important.

Students in my classroom examples above would learn more easily if they found a sense of community. Communal truth-creation experiences stimulate complex Postformal Thought (see earlier section). In the psychology of aging class example, students found community by hearing the from-the-heart story of the struggles of their fellow student and by having a chance to talk about it. The desire to synthesize, ask questions, and generally learn more followed feelings of community. There were fewer feelings of marginality and more feelings of mattering to each other. Complex Postformal Thought developed, with participants rising to a higher level of analysis and logic, as the truths of the others in that classroom community challenged the truth of each participant. They cared about the others in the community enough to give it a try and to do the required cognitive work. This serves the learning mission.

Three Sample Approaches

Below are three detailed examples of methods for teaching complex thought in the college classroom, nested in complex postmodern world views and honoring the desire for community (see Sinnott, in preparation b, "Paths to Complex Thought: Tools for Teaching College Students to Think Postformally. The Professor's Guide to Easy-to-Use Methods"). These methods are taken from my psychology classes, but the approach generalizes well to many other settings. In generalizing to "teaching" situations involving clients or patients, the basic principle underlying the method can guide the interaction. Basic principles that are listed at the end of each method might also be applied to a practitioner/client teaching/learning experience. Notice that while the activities may be used for other purposes, here they specifically are used to build the operations of postformal thought. The teacher will continue to build on these operations from class to class.

Method 1. Work in Small Groups: Creating a Grading System for the Semester

This is an activity for the first days of class. It's fun and offers a heady taste of power to students who are accustomed to simply being opposed to professors or submissive to them. While students make decisions about how many points something like the term paper should be worth, they are getting to know each other and beginning to appreciate the fact that evaluation can be accomplished many different ways! Groups for this activity should be small, so that even shy or less articulate students can have their say.

You, the professor, decide the ground rules of the grading system (for example, what the major assignments are). Students decide, by consensus, within your limits, how many points of the total obtainable points any given assignments are worth. It is important for you to have some nonnegotiable guidelines written in your syllabus to set realistic limits on the discussion. You probably don't want a grading system that gives 100% of the possible points for attendance!

Notice that the idea here is to create community, good process, and "truth" together, honoring each other's standards and beliefs. That central idea applies to the practitioner/client context as well. Creating a treatment regimen is different from creating a grading system, but it can convey the same philosophy and message of personal worth, as well as the complex logical stance that medicine is, after all, both an art and a science in which "truth" is created almost as often as it is revealed in empirical studies.

Postformal thinking operations most enhanced by this method: parameter setting, multiple solutions, multiple methods should be learned during this activity.

Time needed: one to two 50-minute class periods.

Other materials needed: chalkboard or other device for displaying the several grading systems.

Preparations needed—professor: Know your own grading "nonnegotiables"; describe the method to the students; explain why you are letting them help create the system by which they are graded. Perhaps the hardest part is deciding how much latitude you feel comfortable giving students in the decisions about the points each assignment should be worth (which you alone will finally evaluate as to correctness and quality). In a writing course, for example, written assignments might be mandated to receive 50% or more of points. Build these constraints into your syllabus.

Preparations needed—class: The class should be broken down into groups of three to five students (fewer than three cannot challenge each others' ideas; more than five, a dominant student emerges and makes it harder for quiet students to have their say). The class needs to understand that this is a form of the Delphi system (so named because the Greeks consulted an oracle at Delphi to obtain answers to difficult questions). It is a research tool used in long-distance decision making in which consensus must be reached. Successive iterations through the process lead to a consensus decision. Skeptical classes should be made aware that this is not a trick, but a chance to exercise some freedom for a change, and with it, some responsibility. For advanced classes, this exercise provides a chance for students to get a taste of what it's like to be the professor.

End product: a grading system arrived at by consensus, based on professor guidelines (expressed in syllabus), used during the remainder of the course as the professor evaluates quality and correctness of student work.

Another end product is a discussion for you and your students. Students should come to see that there is no one definite authority or one absolute value system that determines the quality of their work in class—at least, until they create one that then becomes the absolute system. They should notice that there are many possible solutions to the problem of creating a grading system, and that there are many ways to get to the same outcome.

Example of use in class: I use this method at the start of undergraduate classes on the psychology of aging. After my preliminary remarks and preliminary syllabus scan, and after students introduce themselves to someone near them they have never met before ("because we're all in this together"), students are placed in groups of five, based on where they happen to be sitting. I ask them to look again at the syllabus and identify the requirements printed there. These usually include quizzes, a term paper, and a 10-minute presentation exploring how aging is portrayed in a movie or other cultural product. I ask them to think about anything else that they want to add to the "requirements" list, leading to a grade in this class. (At this point some winning and losing ideas are offered, and are fun for everyone—for example, "Bringing our grandmothers to class" (loser); "Picking a cross-cultural topic for the term paper" (winner); "interviewing our grandparents using standard questions" (winner); "participation" (winner). (Variations: see below.) I ask them to be scientist-observers of what is happening during this process.

The groups now begin discussion in earnest, while I circulate among them, answering questions and making sure that all students have a chance to speak. Someone in each group is the reporter who will write the group's proposed system on the board for the class to view. When a group has created a point system that includes at least all the requirements stated in the syllabus, the reporter writes it on the board.

When all the systems are on the board open discussion begins. Discussion usually reveals conflicts in values and personal goals, conflicts that can be discussed later in the class in a general way in the context of attitudes toward aging.

Students are now ready to vote on the plans. For simplicity, in this example there are three plans:

Group 1: quizzes, 300 points; term paper, 100 points; presentation, 50 points; interview, 50 points.

Group 2: quizzes, 150 points; term paper, 200 points; presentation, 100 points; interview, 50 points.

Group 3: quizzes 200 points; term paper, 200 points; presentation, 100 points.

Since there is no overall agreement, we need to discuss and vote on things requirement by requirement. Starting with quizzes, pointing out that we must reach consensus and a total of 500 points, I ask for a class show of hands as to whether they can settle for 300 points for quizzes; 200 points; 100 points. If no consensus can be reached, we go on to the next requirement, term paper, following the same system of voting. Eventually some systems are modified and consensus is obtained. I find that starting with the requirement on which there already is some consensus (like the term paper, above) puts students in a consensus mindset and speeds things up. If a stalemate is reached, and if discussion won't help, students go back to small groups to work out a whole new set of points. They have, however, been influenced by the earlier iterations and discussions, so views of what should happen begin to converge over time.

When a system is finally in place it may not look at all like the original ones:

Final system: quizzes, 250 points; term paper, 150 points; presentation, 35 points; interview, 65 points.

Discussion may follow on the variant activities and on the consensus task. See discussion questions below.

General steps to use this method in any class:

1. Divide students into groups of three to five persons.
2. Ask each group to reach consensus within their group about the number of points each required activity should earn, adding extra requirements as they see fit.
3. Direct each group to then write their plan on the board.
4. Conduct a general discussion of the plans.
5. Hold a vote on the points for each requirement, by requirement, e.g., "the term paper." Simple majority wins.
6. If a stalemate occurs, send the students back to small groups to create a new plan, and have them revise postings on board.
7. Continue until overall consensus is reached.
8. If no further discussion, enter the final point system is entered on each student's syllabus, and on yours, to be followed during the course of the semester.

Possible pitfalls/problems:

1. Students are not reaching consensus! Solution: This fear has never become a reality in my 20 plus years of using this method. The solution is a simple one: tell them you are willing to wait as long as it takes for consensus to form. Then do so. It helps to explain that this difficult consensus building is the challenge of democracy, of research teams, of work groups, or of adulthood, so their practice here in class will be very helpful in real life.
2. One student tries to dominate a group's discussion. Solution: assign roles to members of the group. One person makes sure that everyone has a chance to contribute, says "Time's up" when someone has spoken for a stated period of time, and passes the right to speak to the next group member. If this does not work, you can stay with that group and play the timekeeper role yourself.

3. The group plans are so widely divergent that no one plan gets a majority. Solution: send everyone back into discussion groups to create a brand-new plan.
4. A month later students want to create a new grading system. A student joins the class a week late and wants to have a say in the grading system. Solution: just say no, based on the ground rules.

Discussion questions:

1. Did you miss having an authority decide for you? Why? Now that we have reached a decision, do you miss having an authority decide? What changed?
2. What "really" happened during this exercise (used with the variation; see below)?
3. Could you solve this problem without setting ground rules beyond what is in the syllabus?
4. Is this data analyzable without setting parameters (used with the variant; see below)?
5. Was there only one solution to this problem? Can you think of other situations in which there would be more than one solution to a problem?
6. We all concluded that the term paper (alter this to suit what happened in your class) should be worth the most points, but different groups got there using different plans. What were two different paths by which a group concluded that the term paper should be worth the most points?

Variations: Students might be asked to observe the most important things that happen during this activity. These data may be used for analysis and transformed into the basis for future research. The qualitative data might also be used to demonstrate that the "lenses" of each researcher are different, and by extension, that different versions of "truth" and "reality" can emerge from intelligent viewers analyzing the same events.

General principle: Truth is a cocreation.

Method 2. Work in Small Groups: Being a Lawyer for the Prosecution and the Defense

This exercise is useful whenever there is a topic that can be analyzed from two different perspectives. Since that description includes most of the topics that come up in the university setting, this exercise is useful in a wide variety of classes! In the early stages of a class, students might simply be contrasting a couple of concepts. Later in the class they might bring larger bodies of information to bear on the question of which is the best (i.e., most useful) way to see a problem. At the end of a class, arguing the differing positions might form a capstone experience. Classes from different disciplines might even argue differing sides of the "case." The goals are mastery and logical application of the class material, learning to cite scholarly sources, and learning to critique logical arguments.

Why is this activity couched in terms of the courtroom, "lawyers for the prosecution and the defense"? Just because it's more fun and realistic that way! Students have seen some courtroom-related TV shows, and, unfortunately, a certain number have been in court themselves. As experts in their chosen fields of study they may be expert witnesses in a courtroom some day. And the news is full of notorious, historic, and ordinary court cases. So the activity seems professional and entertaining at the same time.

When using this activity it helps to contextualize it in terms of a reasonably current and interesting news event. As you'll see in my example below, I take advantage of the actual occurrence of a fiery train wreck that took place not too far from our campus and involved residents of a nearby community. It also helps motivation that in the case of the train wreck an actual lawsuit is involved. In the United States at this time in history, almost any newsworthy event involves a lawsuit, so providing a "real-life" case is an easy goal to attain.

One advantage of using this "making a case" method is that it makes it very clear that an *argument* is based on *available* facts, and as such is fallible, not a "God's eye view" of truth. The use of a courtroom metaphor also suggests that, although we can't achieve that "God's eye view," we still must decide about truth in the best way we can, and, having decided, go on with life. In this way court experiences mimic the experience of complex postformal thinking with its decisions about reality that are based on necessary subjectivity and commitment to a choice of logics. These points about thinking can be reinforced in class after the "court battle" is over.

Postformal thinking operations most enhanced by this method: metatheory shift, problem definition, parameter setting, pragmatism, paradox.

Time needed: one 50-minute class period; two class periods if improvement in expository writing is an additional goal.

Other materials needed: chalkboard or other device for displaying information about the events of the "case" that forms the basis of the activity.

Preparations needed—professor: Learn enough about the real case that you can tell a lively story about it! Student involvement is enhanced when you can provide those extra details in response to questions. If this was a real court case it helps to know how it was decided, so that you can communicate that decision after the class work is done. This helps keep the students who are still concrete or formal thinkers interested and involved. It is important to let students know, however, that, although a case is decided in a particular way, this does not mean that the arguments of the side that won were necessarily better! Other factors might come into play in a court situation.

Preparations needed—class: The class should be broken down into groups of three to five students, and students should have been told to bring whatever reference materials are needed such as the textbook, if those are needed or permitted to build their best cases.

End product: a summary of the best case (composite of the several groups' cases) for the "prosecution" and the best case for the "defense." Students may then secretly vote on which case they think was more logically and factually meritorious. Students may be informed of the actual court decision, and its basis in logic and fact, if this is known. The ultimate "end product" is mastery and appropriate application of the class material.

Example of use in class: I last used this method in my Midlife Development class, an undergraduate developmental psychology course in which students examine changes that occur between the ages of 20 and 60, especially changes and roles related to age. The class had been studying sensory and intellectual changes during those years, and I had stressed two chapters in the textbook in particular on those topics.

I introduced the activity by telling the true story of a train wreck that took place near our university, a wreck that involved two men who resided in the suburbs nearby. As I told the story I drew diagrams to illustrate parts of it on the board. I can assure you that the story is very dramatic (much more so than you might guess from reading the bare outline here) and that (what a rare event!) not one student in the entire history of the class has ever lost interest during the telling of the story.

Late in the evening of the night of the biggest, most blinding blizzard of the year, two trains approached each other head on, too fast, on the same track. They were a commuter train and a freight train that also had a few passenger cars. They crashed and a huge fire was ignited from the spilled fuel. Eleven persons, most of them young, burned to death, trapped in the cars, which had emergency exits neither they nor emergency crews could open. The two local men were part of the crew running those trains, and they were middle-aged.

The ashes from the fire were still warm when litigation began. Among those being sued were the track maintenance company, the company running the commuter train, the company running the freight train, emergency rescue crews, insurance companies, and the train crews (or their families, if deceased). The portion of the litigation for which the class might act as expert witness is the lawsuit against the two middle-aged men running the commuter train in which they and others died. These two were in charge, responsible for the operation of the commuter train, which was found to have been going faster than it should have been going. The argument could be made that they were not competent to run the train at this time due to problems of sensory change or intellectual slowing. (Of course, if the men were the cause of the accident either by virtue of aging-related factors or general negligence, the insurance and other companies would be less liable. The motivation of the prosecution to prove this was high! And demonstrating that age-related factors were implicated in the men causing the wreck would have large ramifications for hiring and employment.)

I answered as many questions as the class wanted me to after I finished relating the details of the case, and continued to do so as the groups worked together. The class divided into groups and each group was assigned the task of making the expert case for either the defense or the prosecution, using studies and data from the chapters in our text. Roaming among groups let me correct common problems such as misinterpretations of the general statement that "sensory acuity lessens with age." That general research finding, when you look at the studies themselves, usually means the investigator tested respondents from age 20 through age 80. So, at what point, and how much, does sensory acuity drop, as "demonstrated by the research"? The answer to this question is important for this trial situation. Seeing the distinction is important for students' logical and critical thinking. They need to understand that research findings are limited by their contexts and are subject to interpretation.

Another common error that offers an opportunity to teach critical thinking is students trying to figure out what did cause the accident (a worthy question), so much so that they forget to focus on the case they are trying to build as hired expert psychologist witnesses. For example, students might want to vehemently argue that the accident was caused by the snow. But it is less valuable for a psychology expert witness to argue that the accident was really caused by the snow, and therefore that the men were not guilty of it, than to argue that the men were not likely to be incompetent in using their senses or intelligence, as the prosecution might suggest they are, because psychological research does not support incompetence in those areas for this age group. Keep focusing on the logical case you are trying to build!

Students working in groups created their best cases. They offered them to the class. The class critiqued the logic, then combined the best features, of all the defense cases and all the prosecution cases. Class members secretly voted for the side they believed made the overall best psychology expert case. (This provides a good chance in class to discuss the differences between "making the best case," and "my gut-level feeling about this matter.") Students voted that the defense made the best case (i.e., that the men were not responsible due to age-related factors). I then told the class the outcome: that a court had eventually ruled that the two men were generally negligent but not at fault for age-related reasons (which would have had an impact on hiring and work practices), and that other companies were found to be liable as well.

Students were able to take their improved (after class discussion) prosecution/defense case home, make it even better, write it out as well as they could, and turn it in during the next class for some possible points, based on its quality.

General steps to use this method in any class:

1. Tell the story, concluding with the courtroom context and the students' roles as expert witnesses. Who is suing whom about what?
2. Divide students into groups of three to five students each. Select the group member who will report the final results to the class.

3. Assign half the groups to build a logical case for the "prosecution" based on your choice of reference materials, the other half to do the same for the "defense."
4. Remind the students to build logical arguments using information cited (page number in text? investigator name?) and credited to a professional source. (You may wish to help students decide whether the source is a worthy one as you go from group to group answering questions.)
5. Let student groups build their cases. Some groups assign a particular person to gather information about each specific aspect of the argument they wish to make. Others work together on all parts of the argument.
6. Have the students report the results and critique the logic of the arguments presented.
7. Direct the students to put the best argument together for "defense" and "prosecution," and report their results.
8. Have the students secretly vote on which of the two arguments carries the most weight, report that result.
9. Tell what was decided in the real-world setting.

Possible pitfalls/problems:

1. No consensus, or one student dominates discussion. Solution: see the discussion under method 1, above.
2. Students want to base their argument on "what's fair" rather than on the logical arguments derived from facts in their resource materials. Solution: explain that, while expert witnesses might be motivated by fairness questions, courts only accept logically prepared factually based arguments. So citing authorities and facts is the way to go here. This is a good chance for students to learn the difference between emotion-based and fact-based arguments. It allows students to learn that in the "real world" of a courtroom it does little good on a practical level to be "right" if you can't get facts lined up to support you. This activity demonstrates how to create a "better" (more compelling) logical case for a position, and how to use the text or other materials for something other than passing exams. It may motivate some students to do research in areas where "it is obvious" that certain things are true, but since no research has been done, no authoritative argument can be made!

Discussion questions:

1. What would make this argument better for these purposes?
2. Although we know that facts about the litigated situation might possibly be determined, is it possible that both sides (prosecution/defense) might make

equally good arguments and offer equally good interpretations of the facts, based on information in your resource materials?

3. Might a court be prejudiced toward one side of the argument simply because more facts can be gathered from these resource materials to support that side?

4. How did you decide how to frame your argument?

5. How did you decide what to include and exclude in building your case?

6. Find a weakness in your argument, or in the argument of the "other side." Is it a weakness because it does not support the case, because it is factually incorrect (based on the resource material), or because it has not been argued in a persuasive way?

7. Do you see any element of paradox in the legal process given the motto: "Let justice prevail"?

8. Does arguing both sides lead to a better understanding of "truth," or simply to cynicism?

Variations: Students might present the oral debate of these two sides of the argument. If this assignment is to be worked into a writing course format, drafts of the final arguments for prosecution or defense might focus on the following: logic, flow of the prose, selection of resource material elements that most strongly support the case, and elegance of presentation of the final argument, buttressed by examples. Even if this is not done in class, students might be told to take their arguments home and, as individuals or teams, perfect either the argument or the expression of it, turning it in later for a grade. You can come back to these arguments later in the semester when you have more resource material that could shed light on the case. For example, when we get to the "Stress" chapter, we can examine another argument (that stressed-out employees caused the train wreck) based on the additional stress information.

General principle: Arguing the point of view of the other side leads to increased abstract and interpersonal understanding and cognitive growth.

Method 3. Work in Small Groups: Data Gathering— What Happened Here?

In most classes students act as *consumers* of information. (Clients are forced into the role of consumers most of the time.) They hear about the area of study in lectures. They read about the area of study in textbooks or journal articles. But some students want to become active professionals in the area of study. Some plan to continue their training with a masters and doctorate. For most areas of study this means, among other things, being a producer of information as well as a consumer of it. Information gathering, or "research" in its many forms, puts the students in a different place in regard to knowledge, and gives them greater power. Armed with a fresh perspective and increased capability, students are in a perfect position to begin to ask questions about the strengths, limits, and contexts of the known. This assists their complex thinking development and turns them into informed, critical consumers of the information produced by other data gatherers in their field.

In this activity the class takes a try at being producers of information. In the process they learn that all information is viewed through lenses that alter the way information is known. They also learn some of the basic pitfalls that make the gathering of information more difficult than it first seems to be.

This activity is informal, deliberately. The goal of this activity is for the student to begin to look more closely at the world, at theories, and at all knowledge and thereby gain a more realistic idea of the inherent strengths and limitations of our understanding. Becoming aware of this basic epistemological problem usually results in the students' putting the information in your lectures and in the textbook into a different light. Beware! Discussions and critiques might occur!

Because this set of skills is so crucial to critical thinking I have provided two examples below.

Postformal thinking operations most enhanced by this method: metatheory shift, problem definition, process/product shift, parameter setting, multiple solutions, pragmatism, multiple causality, multiple methods, paradox.

Time needed: at least one class period.

Other materials needed: As you'll see from the two class examples below, the "materials" you might use for this activity are limited only by your imagination and creativity. Yet in every case you will need papers and pencils (or other devices for recording information, such as a video camera or computers). You also will need some part of the "real world" to observe (ranging in complexity from crowd behavior at the inauguration of a president to behaviors such as the thoughts that float through your consciousness in a dark, quiet room where you sit alone). Students might want to use calculators for simple data analyses. Some device (e.g., chalkboard, overhead projector) for displaying the results to the class, for discussion, usually comes in handy.

Preparations needed—professor: If you are sending a class to a public place to observe, make sure they won't encounter people who will be frightened or annoyed by their behavior or their mere presence. (In my more naïve youth I once sent a student group to observe day versus night parking behavior in a campus parking garage. Six casually dressed young persons, shuffling around the garage at 10:00 P.M., staring and taking notes, looked suspicious. Fear prompted someone to call the police about a possible auto theft gang. When the squad cars pulled up and police surrounded them the students became upset; and so did I when I had to straighten the whole thing out!)

Preparations needed—class: The class should be broken down into groups of three to five students and each group should have data-recording materials. The activity should be connected to some class topic about which the students have already read.

End product: There will be several sets of results, as the data are more deeply analyzed. The real "end product" is a better sense of how information is produced and how theories come into being. Another "end product" is a better sense of how to ask questions about the strengths and the inevitable weaknesses of the data.

First example of use in class—getting to know you: This activity works well toward the beginning of any of my undergraduate psychology courses, a point at which we review some general methods in behavioral science research. I tell the class that I have five questions for them to answer using any method they think is valid and feasible in a short time. Here are the five questions, which they write down: (1) How many people here like tofu? (2) Do you know what tofu is? (3) What is the favorite clothing color of undergraduates? (4) Does anyone in class know a joke related to Cleveland (which happens to be my hometown)? (5) What proportion of people in the room have done research? At that point I step back and to the side of the room and wait.

At first there is a moment, several, actually, of silence. Undergraduates have not been taught to take the initiative! When they realize that nothing is going to happen until they do something themselves (a valuable lesson in its own right), either some brave student will step up to organize things, or several subgroups with leaders will begin to organize things. The single or the several group leaders will begin to read out the questions, doing a hand count in a less-than-organized way. When they have answered the questions in some fashion, students again turn to me with satisfaction. They have answers.

The catch is that we are about to discover four important things. The research answer you get depends on how you frame (contextualize) the question. The information you get depends on the respondents' understanding of the terms in the questions. Statistics and "results" are distorted by the kinds of numbers you can produce from the answers to the questions. And, who you choose to be part of the sample has a bearing on the results. Understanding these key things about context and lenses is important to understanding scientific and other research. Any of these ideas can be considered in the context of any of the five questions. If a class is having a problem getting one particular concept, you might want to work with it using all five.

So we start with question 1. The leader reads the question, and I ask if anyone has written something slightly different down. For example, the leader may read "How many in class like tofu?" (answer: 2) while someone else has written down "Do most people like tofu?" (answer: 2/28, therefore "no"). We consider the different answers that might emerge from the two different questions, and how the answers might be phrased. We consider how many possible ways there are to express a question related to the liking of tofu, all of them pertinent, but each leading to a differently nuanced data set. Did all the respondents understand the terms of the question?

Who is in the sample? As I originally stated the question "How many people here like tofu?" the sample should have been everyone "here" (which is a classroom), and that includes me, the instructor. But every time (and here is a lesson for those of us who teach in order to be noticed), *they fail to count me, although my hand is up!* Again, the point is not to induce guilt in the students for ignoring the professor but to get them to reflect on the biases we bring as researchers, biases that distort "knowledge" by distorting (in this case) the sample. (This becomes especially apparent in the follow-up to the "Cleveland joke" question, which calls for a yes/no response. Having grown up in Cleveland, I do know a Cleveland joke. I even am permitted under rules of political correctness to tell the Cleveland joke, though I seldom do. But no one else in the class ever knows a Cleveland joke. So this leads to an answer of "No," if students are the entire sample, and "Yes" if I am in the sample, two different answers to our research question.)

We move on to question 2, "Do you know what tofu is?" Again I ask for variants in the written form of the research question, variants that might distort the results. For example, if a student hears the word "you" to mean "you, singular" he or she answers differently from a student would get if the word was heard as plural. Usually there turn out to be quite a few students who have no idea what tofu is. This gives me a chance to ask whether the order of the research questions matters. Does it make more sense to ask the "know" question first, then ask the "like" question only to those respondents who know what tofu is? Which of the respondents who said they liked it said so in the abstract, without ever tasting it, and which have really tasted it and like it?

It depends what you want to know! Let's go back to the "do you understand the question" issue. Do you want to know who already likes it (perhaps in the context of a marketing study of who will buy it tomorrow) or who needs more information about tofu (so that you can educate them before you market to them next year)? In the first marketing study you need not care if the respondents know what tofu is. Your question about whether they buy it tomorrow will be answered since, if they don't even know what it is, they don't like it yet and are very unlikely to buy it. At bottom, the question-ordering issue becomes a sampling issue if you only want those who answered a certain way on a prior question to go on.

Question 3: "What is the favorite clothing color of undergraduates?" This one is also ripe for many interpretations, each of which changes the type of data needed and obtained. Most times students try to answer this one by looking at what classmates are wearing, or by naming their own favorite clothing colors in descending order of preference and seeing if others agree. I point out the biases of these two approaches. They come up with other approaches, and I point out the biases of each of those, too. Eventually we agree on the general rule that "Since all approaches are biased, each in a different way, the best you can do is consciously select the bias you prefer." Going on to the type of answer demanded, note that only the favorite color is requested. So knowing the range of preferred colors is unnecessary to answer the question. Finally, in terms of sampling, we notice that the question refers to undergraduates as a whole. Is our class representative of all undergraduates? Can we answer the question at all, or, if we choose to use the data from outside class, to whom do the results generalize?

Question 4: the Cleveland joke question. By this time their world view has been rather challenged and they are tiring, so the main purpose of this question (and the last one) is to reinforce the issues already mentioned above. Who is in the sample? What is a joke understood to be? Must they tell the joke to prove that they know it? Is the answer to be in Yes/No, or count or proportion, format?

Finally, Question 5: "What percentage of people in the room have done research?" This is a light way to finish up this activity, since we know the sample, and the meanings, except for the meaning of "have done research." Students still wrestling with the sense of awe in which they hold the research enterprise overlook the fact that everyone in the classroom has just done research! The answer is 100%. Although we have done very low-level research, students usually feel empowered that they have done any research at all.

The activity ends with my recapping the four basic things we have observed about the difficulties in gathering knowledge and in knowing anything objectively. They will be asked on a quiz to describe the four and to illustrate those principles with examples from our class exercise. Best of all, feelings of community will have been facilitated.

Second example of use in class—door-opening behavior: The second class example shows how the above technique can be used during class time, but outside of the classroom setting. Many of the points made under the first example above can be made again in this activity, but I have not repeated them here. The goals are to understand the partially constructed nature of truth and the ordinary challenges of knowing anything as purely objective truth.

The class is told they will be observing behavior, namely door-opening behavior. What do people do when there is the opportunity to open or hold the door for each other? Students are told that they will do this research in groups. Each group will have to decide the specific topic of the observation, the hypothesis that they are trying to support, and how data will be collected over a five-minute period of observation. After a few minutes of planning, the groups go to their vantage points to watch people open/not open, hold/not hold doors for each other.

When the observation is completed and the groups return to the classroom, they summarize results of their studies. Some of my initial questions include: What did you see happening? Was your hypothesis supported? What numbers did you gather that seem to show this? Additional questions can be added, of course.

As the class describes and discusses groups' results it becomes clear that individuals in the group, all attempting to record the same types of things, "see" different things, all of which are "really" happening! Groups "discover" the four important things (discussed above) by doing this exercise:

1. The research answer you get depends on how you frame (context) the question. For example, was the question about holding doors or opening doors? Maybe the observed hold doors often, but never open them for another person, giving the answers "yes" *and* "no" to the question "are students polite?"

2. The information you get depends on the respondents' (observers') understanding of the terms in the questions. For example, what does "opening" mean in practice? If one observer thinks it means "grabbing the handle, pulling it open, and holding the door until the person goes through it" and another observer thinks it means "pulling the door open, then letting it go" the two observers might have very different data!

3. Statistics and "results" are distorted by the kinds of numbers you can produce from the answers to the questions. For example, some students produce "yes/no" (nominal scale) answers to their research questions about door opening; others produce "number of times" or "how long" (ratio scale) answers. Sometimes both kinds of answers occur in the same group watching the same events, trying to support the same hypotheses! The yes/no data might suggest a different "truth" about the relationship between door holding and time of day than "how long" data does: students might hold the door for another both early in the day and late in the day, but they hold the door much longer early in the day!

4. Who you chose to be part of the sample affects the results. For example, once one of my research groups watched all students while another (at the same spot) watched males holding doors for others. The former found that students did open doors for others, while the latter found that they did not. What to make of this? Upon further research, we determined that both sets of results were correct since females hold doors much more than males do and "all students" included lots of females.

General Steps to Use This Method in Any Class:

1. Give students fairly simple research questions to answer, questions that can be interpreted/heard in more than one way.
2. Instruct individuals or groups of students to answer the questions by any means they jointly choose.
3. Have the students examine the data obtained by each group.
4. Note the uncertain parts of operational definitions and the choices of number systems.

5. Mention alternative ways to operationally define, score, or interpret.
6. Direct the students to use uncertainties as leads to future research.
7. Direct them to use the results across groups/individuals to do a meta-analysis of findings.
8. Direct them to use contradictions in the results across groups/individuals as leads to future research hypotheses.
9. Discuss the nature of "truth" and "knowing" and the way multiple (flawed) studies lead to better research and theories.
10. Discuss why "two heads are better than one."

Possible pitfalls/problems:

1. Some students may feel lost without someone telling them what to do and how to do it. Nurture these people! Ask them to suspend judgment and to try to tolerate their discomfort until they can appreciate where this exercise is going!
2. An infrequent problem: some people being observed (or close to those being observed) get angry about "being observed." For example, a cashier in our campus ice cream snack shop has barely begun to speak to me when I pay her—after 15 years of silence. The reason? She was in the line of sight one semester long ago when students were observing "who bought what kind of food." She didn't like them looking at her (even though they were really looking at the food). So, try to keep students away from sensitive people.

Discussion questions: These have been mentioned in the examples above, and in the list of "general steps" for using the method.

Variations: These involve variations on the original research question. Consequently, they are almost infinite! Any fairly ambiguous question that might be heard different ways, with answers that might be tallied using a variety of number systems will do.

General principle: The details of one's approach to a problem or a patient affects the outcome.

Conclusion: Relevance to Healthcare Providers

Teaching the Next Generation of Providers

In this chapter I have attempted to share a little about the evolution of my teaching as a professor, some theoretical background related to my expanded style of teaching, and some sample methods for working in a different way in a classroom environment. My hope is to give you, as a practitioner training future practitioners, some potentially helpful ideas about teaching in context. The ideas summarized here are directed toward viewing teaching as "nourishment for life" of whole students, in context. The context is that of the larger world but also of the student who has a mind, a heart, a spirit, a body, and a need for community. We can prepare students for jobs as professionals while also honoring them as whole human beings with complex lives. In the classroom context the relevance of the comments in this chapter is very clear.

"Teaching" (and Learning From) Patients

The second purpose of this chapter is to offer ideas for a potentially expanded view of teaching as it pertains to the relationship of a practitioner "educating" a patient or client. While we might not readily think of this interaction as "teaching" in the traditional sense, it is just that. This means that the views and attitudes we bring to the encounter with that client can be modified by the ideas expressed in this chapter so that the whole of the client might be honored in our encounter and so that our teaching might be more effective. Imagine a simple example. Would it be more effective to lecture a patient on a particular drug regimen, or method of cleaning a catheter, or would it be more effective (after giving the basic information) to ask the patient how he or she will work this regimen into daily life? Wouldn't it be helpful to ask how doing this medical thing makes the patient feel, or might affect his or her intimate partner relationship? We know the answer, from experience and from our own desires as future patients. Respect and dialogue always win the day and make for more effective learning. We want to be part of a community that is a healing one.

If you find some value in these ideas, incorporate them into your work as a teaching professional. And, as a learner (which we forever are), make each learning situation nourishment for your life, whatever the skill of your teachers.

References

Hofstadter, D. R. (1979). *Gödel, Escher, Bach: An eternal golden braid.* New York: Basic Books.

Inhelder, B., & Piaget, J. (1958). *The growth of logical thinking from childhood to adolescence: An essay on the construction of formal operations structures.* (A. Parsons & S. Milgram, Trans.). New York: Basic Books. (Original French work published in 1955.)

Kahaney, P., Janangelo, J., & Perry, L. A. M. (Eds.). (1993). *Theoretical and critical perspectives on teacher change.* Norwood, NJ: Ablex.

Kegan, R. (1982). *The evolving self: Problem and process in human development.* Cambridge, MA: Harvard University Press.

Mezirow, J. (2000). *Learning as transformation: Critical perspectives on a theory in process.* San Francisco: Jossey-Bass.

Perry, W. G. (1970). *Forms of ethical and intellectual development in the college years: A scheme.* New York: Holt, Rinehart & Winston.

Pipher, M. B. (1999). *Another country: Navigating the emotional terrain of our elders.* New York: Riverhead Books.

Sinnott, J. D. (1981). The theory of relativity: A metatheory for development? *Human Development, 24,* 293–311.

Sinnott, J. D. (1984). Postformal reasoning: The relativistic stage. In M. L. Commons, F. A. Richards & C. Armon (Eds.), *Beyond formal operations: Late adolescent and adult cognitive development.* New York: Praeger.

Sinnott, J. D. (1989). Lifespan relativistic Postformal Thought. In M. L. Commons, J. D. Sinnott, F. A. Richards, & C. Armon (Eds.), *Beyond formal operations I.* New York: Praeger.

Sinnott, J. D. (1990). Yes, it's worth the trouble! Unique contributions from everyday cognition studies. Paper presented at the Twelfth West Virginia University Conference on Lifespan Developmental Psychology: Mechanisms of Everyday Cognition, Morgantown, WV.

Sinnott, J. D. (1991a). What do we do to help John? A case study of everyday problem solving in a family making decisions about an acutely psychotic member. In J. D. Sinnott & J. C. Cavanaugh (Eds.), *Bridging paradigms: Positive development in adulthood and cognitive aging.* New York: Praeger.

Sinnott, J. D. (1991b). Limits to problem solving: Emotion, intention, goal clarity, health, and other factors in postformal thought. In J. D. Sinnott & J. C. Cavanaugh (Eds.), *Bridging paradigms: Positive development in adulthood and cognitive aging.* New York: Praeger.

Sinnott, J. D. (1993a). Teaching in a chaotic new physics world: Teaching as a dialogue with reality. In P. Kahaney, J. Janangelo, & L. A. M. Perry (Eds.), *Theoretical and critical perspectives on teacher change.* Norwood, NJ: Ablex.

Sinnott J. D. (1993b). Use of complex thought and resolving intragroup conflicts: A means to conscious adult development in the workplace. In J. Demick & P. M. Miller (Eds.), *Development in the workplace.* Hillsdale, NJ: L. Erlbaum.

Sinnott, J. D. (1994a). Development and yearning: Cognitive aspects of spiritual development. *Journal of Adult Development, 1*(2), 91–99.

Sinnott, J. D. (1994b). (Ed.) *Interdisciplinary handbook of adult lifespan learning.* Westport, CT: Greenwood.

Sinnott, J. D. (1996). The development of complex reasoning: Postformal Thought. In F. Blanchard-Fields & T. M. Hess (Eds.), *Perspectives on cognitive change in adulthood and aging.* New York: McGraw-Hill.

Sinnott, J. D. (1997). Brief report: Complex Postformal Thought in skilled research administrators. *Journal of Adult Development, 4*(1), 45–53.

Sinnott, J. D. (1998a). Creativity and Postformal Thought. In C. E. Adams-Price (Ed.), *Creativity and aging: Theoretical and empirical approaches.* New York: Springer.

Sinnott, J. D. (1998b). *The development of logic in adulthood: Postformal Thought and its applications.* (Plenum Series on Adult Development, J. Demick, Ed.). New York: Plenum.

Sinnott, J. D. (2000). Cognitive aspects of unitative states: Spiritual self-realization, intimacy, and knowing the unknowable. In M. E. Miller & A. N. West (Eds.), *Spirituality, ethics, and relationship in adulthood: Clinical and theoretical explorations.* Madison, CT: Psychosocial Press.

Sinnott, J. D. (2002). Postformal Thought and adult development: Living in balance. In J. Demick and C. Andreoletti (Eds.), *Handbook of adult development.* New York: Plenum.

Sinnott, J. D. (in preparation, a). *Moving toward love: Creating community in a global society.*

Sinnott, J. D. (in preparation, b). *Workbook for teaching postformal complex thought in the university classroom.*

Sinnott, J. D., & Cavanaugh, J. C. (Eds.) (1991). *Bridging paradigms: Positive development in adulthood and cognitive aging.* New York: Praeger.

Sinnott, J. D., & Johnson, L. (1996a). *Reinventing the university: A radical proposal for a problem focused university.* Norwood, NJ: Ablex.

Sinnott, J. D., & Johnson, L. (1996b). Reinventing the university: A reasonable proposal for a problem-focused university for the 21st century. *Futures Research Quarterly 12*, (4), 61–69.

Wolf, F. A. (1981). *Taking the quantum leap: The new physics for nonscientists.* San Francisco: Harper & Row.

For Further Reading

Offering additional references related to the Theory of Postformal Thought, New Physics Theory, Chaos Theory, General Systems Theory, Humanistic/Transpersonal Psychology, and Theories of Self-Organizing Systems

Abraham, R. (1985). Is there chaos without noise? In P. Fisher & W. R. Smith (Eds.), *Chaos, fractals, and dynamics.* New York: M. Dekker.

Alper, J. (1989). The chaotic brain: New models of behavior. *Psychology Today, 23,* 21.

Barton, S. (1994). Chaos, self organization, and psychology. *American Psychologist, 49,* (1) 5–14.

Bohm, D. (1980). *Wholeness and the implicate order.* London: Routledge & Kegan Paul.

Bronowski, J. (1974). *The ascent of man.* Boston, Little Brown.

Capra, F. (1974). *The tao of physics: An exploration of the parallels between modern physics and Eastern mysticism.* Berkeley, CA: Shambhala.

Cassirer, E. (1950). *The problem of knowledge: Philosphy, science, and history since Hegel.* (W. H. Woglom & C. W. Hendel, Trans.). New Haven, CT: Yale University Press. (Original German work published in 1906.)

Cassirer, E. (1953). *Substance and function, and Einstein's theory of relativity.* (W. C. Swabey & M. C. Swabey, Trans.). New York: Dover. (Original German work published in 1910 and 1921.)

Cassirer, E. (1956). *Determinism and indeterminism in modern physics: Historical and systematic studies of the problem of causality.* (O. T. Benfey, Trans.). New Haven, CT: Yale University Press. (Original German work published in 1937.)

Cavanaugh, J. C. (1989). The utility of concepts in chaos theory for psychological theory and research. Paper presented at the Fourth Adult Development Conference at Harvard University, Cambridge MA.

Cavanaugh, J. C., & McGuire, L. (1994). The chaos of lifespan learning. In J. D. Sinnott (Ed.), *Interdisciplinary handbook of adult lifespan learning.* Westport, CT: Greenwood.

Crutchfield, J. P., Farmer, J. D., Packard, N. H., & Shaw, R. S. (1986). Chaos. *Scientific American, 255*(6), 46–57.

Davies, P. C. W. (1989). *The new physics.* New York: Cambridge University Press.

Devaney, R. L. (1989). *An introduction to chaotic dynamical systems.* Redwood City, CA: Addison-Wesley.

Einstein, A. (1961). *Relativity: The special and general theory.* (R. W. Lawson, Trans.) New York: Crown. (Original German works published in 1905 and 1916 respectively.)

Ferguson, M. (1980). *The aquarian conspiracy: Personal and social transformation in the 1980s.* Los Angeles, CA: J. P. Tarcher.

Ford, D. H., & Ford, M. E. (Eds.). (1987). *Humans as self-constructing living systems: Putting the framework to work.* Hillsdale, NJ: L. Erlbaum.

Frankl, V. E. (1963). *Man's search for meaning: An introduction to logotherapy.* (I. Lasch, Trans.). New York: Washington Square Press. (Original German work published in 1946.)

Gleick, J. (1987). *Chaos: Making a new science.* New York: Viking.

Goerner, S. J. (1994). *Chaos and the evolving psychological universe.* Langhorne, PA: Gordon & Breach.

Goldstein, J. (1994). *The unshackled organization.* Portland, OR: Productivity Press.

Gottman, J. (1991). Chaos and regulated change in families: A metaphor for the study of transitions. In P. A. Cohen and E. M. Hetherington (Eds.), *Family transitions.* Hillsdale, NJ: L. Erlbaum.

Kauffman, S. A. (1993). *The origins of order: Self-organization and selection in evolution.* New York: Oxford University Press.

Kelly, K. (1994). *Out of control: The new biology of machines, social systems and the economic world.* Reading, MA: Perseus.

Kramer, D. A. (1983). Postformal operations? A need for further conceptualization. *Human Development, 26,* 91–105.

Labouvie-Vief, G. (1984). Logic and self regulation from youth to maturity: A model. In M. L. Commons, F. A. Richards, & C. Armon (Eds.), *Beyond formal operations: Late adolescent and adult cognitive development.* New York: Praeger.

Labouvie-Vief, G. (1987). *Speaking about feelings:Symbolization and self regulation throughout the life span.* Paper presented at the Third Beyond Formal Operations Conference at Harvard University, Cambridge, MA.

Labouvie-Vief, G. (1992). A neo-Piagetian perspective on adult cognitive development. In R. J. Sternberg and C. A. Berg (Eds.), *Intellectual development.* New York: Cambridge University Press.

Labouvie-Vief, G. (1994). *Psyche and eros: Mind and gender in the life course.* Cambridge, UK: Cambridge University Press.

Levine, R. L., & Fitzgerald, H. E. (Eds.) (1992). *Analysis of dynamic psychological systems, Vols. 1 & 2.* New York: Plenum.

Lock Land, G. T. (1973). *Grow or die: The unifying principle of transformation.* New York: Random House.

Lorenz, E. N. (1963). Deterministic nonperiodic flow. *Journal of Atmospheric Sciences, 20,* 130–141.

Lorenz, E. N. (1979). Predictability: Does the flap of a butterfly's wings in Brazil set off a tornado in Texas? Paper presented at the annual meeting of the American Association for the Advancement of Science, Washington, DC.

Mahoney, M. J. (1991). *Human change processes: The scientific foundations of psychotherapy.* New York: Basic Books.

Maturana, H. R., & Varela, F. J. (1980). *Autopoiesis and cognition: The realization of the living.* Boston: D. Reidel.

Miller, J. G. (1978). *Living systems.* New York: McGraw-Hill.

Nicholis, G., & Prigogene, I. (1989). *Exploring complexity: An introduciton.* New York: W. H. Freeman.

Pool, R. (1989). Is it healthy to be chaotic? *Science, 243,* 604–607.

Prigogene, I., & Stengers, I. (1984). *Order out of chaos: Man's new dialogue with nature.* New York: Bantam.

Russell, B. (1969). *The ABC of relativity.* (Felix Pirani, Ed.). New York: New American Library.

Smith, L. B., & Thelan, E. (Eds.) (1993). *A dynamic systems approach to development: Applications.* Cambridge, MA: MIT Press.

Underwood, P. (1991). *Three strands in the braid: A guide for enablers of learning.* San Anselmo, CA: A Tribe of Two Press.

Von Bertalanffy, L. (1968). *General systems theory: Foundations, development, applications.* New York: Braziller.

Von Neumann, J. & Morgenstern, O. (1947). *Theory of games and economic behavior.* Princeton, NJ: Princeton University Press.

Waldrop, M. M. (1992). *Complexity: The emerging science at the edge of order and chaos.* New York: Simon and Schuster.

Weiner, N. (1961). *Cybernetics, or, Control and communication in the animal and the machine.* Cambridge, MA: MIT Press.

Yan, B. (1995). *Nonabsolute/relativistic (N/R) thinking: A possible unifying commonality underlying models of postformal reasoning.* Unpublished Ph.D. dissertation, University of British Columbia, Vancouver.

Yan, B., & Arlin, P. K. (1995). Nonabsolute/relativistic thinking: A common factor underlying models of postformal reasoning? *Journal of Adult Development, 2*(4), 223–240.

Zukav, G. (1980). *The dancing wu li masters: An overview of the new physics.* New York: Bantam.

Contributors
Index

Contributors

Karin Dahlberg is Professor at Växjö University in Sweden. Her doctorate was in pedagogy and her professorate in health sciences. Her current research explicates phenomenological epistemology for empirical purposes. Central to this approach is a focus on the patients' perspectives in conducting research projects. Dr. Dahlberg and co-authors Dr. Nancy Drew and Dr. Maria Nyström have described the phenomenological research approach in a new book: *Reflective Lifeworld Research* (Sweden: Studentlitteratur, 2001).

Nancy L. Diekelmann is Helen Denne Schulte Professor at the University of Wisconsin–Madison School of Nursing, a fellow in the American Academy of Nursing, past president of the Society for Research in Nursing Education, and chair of the University of Wisconsin–Madison Teaching Academy. A noted authority for her work in nursing education and primary healthcare, Dr. Diekelmann has received two Book of the Year awards from the *American Journal of Nursing* for her textbooks *Primary Health Care of the Well Adult* and *Transforming RN Education: Dialogue and Debate* (co-authored with Marsha L. Rather). She received the National League for Nursing Excellence in Nursing Research Award in 2001. Her current research uses interpretive phenomenology to explicate the narratives of teachers, students, and clinicians in nursing education toward a science of nursing education. Dr. Diekelmann has developed a research-based new pedagogy for nursing education: Narrative Pedagogy. She is co-author with John Diekelmann of a forthcoming book—*Schooling Learning Teaching: Toward a Narrative Pedagogy.*

Margaretha Ekebergh is Assistant Professor at the School of Health Sciences, in Borås, Sweden. She has a doctoral degree in caring science and has developed a model for caring-science didactics. Dr. Ekebergh is manager of the didactic unit at the School of Health Sciences. She is responsible for curriculum and didactic development, and oversees clinical studies within the university diploma program in nursing. She has conducted innovative studies within the nursing education program, such as researching a model for reflective supervision. She has also developed an educational idea for an educational hospital ward.

Morgan Harlow is a member of the Narrative Pedagogy Fuld–grant research team at the University of Wisconsin–Madison School of Nursing. She earned degrees in English and journalism from the University of Wisconsin–Madison, and holds a master of fine arts degree in creative writing from George Mason University. She has published fiction and poetry in *Blue Mesa Review, Controlled Burn: A Northwoods Literary Journal, South Dakota Review,* and other literary journals.

Pamela M. Ironside, PhD, RN, is an Associate Professor in the Department of Nursing and Health at Clarke College in Dubuque, Iowa. She teaches research design, research seminar, nursing theories, perspectives on nursing, and a variety of nursing education courses including curriculum development, instruction, and clinical education. Her current research uses interpretive phenomenology to explicate the lived experiences of teachers, students, and citizens in nursing education as a means of developing site-specific, community-driven pedagogies. She is also using a multimethod approach to evaluate Narrative Pedagogy—an alternative approach for nursing education—in introductory nursing courses. She has published research articles in *Journal of Advanced Nursing, Advances in Nursing Science, Journal of Qualitative Health Research,* and *Nursing and Health Care Perspectives.* She is chair-elect of the Nursing Education Advisory Council of the National League for Nursing and is a member of the National League for Nursing Think Tank on Graduate Education for the Nurse Educator Role.

Kathryn Hopkins Kavanagh is the author of *Promoting Cultural Diversity: Strategies for Health Care Professionals* (with Patricia Kennedy; Newbury Park, CA: Sage, 1992), which remains widely cited and is in its fifth printing. She is otherwise widely published in the fields of both medical anthropology and cross-cultural healthcare. Prepared as a mental health clinical nurse specialist and as a medical anthropologist, she focuses her research attention on issues of diversity, multiculturalism, and ideological influences in healthcare. A tenured faculty member at the University of Maryland for many years, Dr. Kavanagh has also been Director of the Baccalaureate Program on the Navajo and Hopi Reservation with Northern Arizona University. She now devotes most of her time to anthropological research, teaching, and writing.

Rosemary A. McEldowney is a Senior Lecturer in the Graduate School of Nursing and Midwifery at Victoria University of Wellington, New Zealand. She is a Fellow of the College of Nurses Aotearoa New Zealand and was recently voted best supervisor by postgraduate students in the Faculty of Humanities and Social Sciences at Victoria University of Wellington. For the past 15 years she has been in the forefront of developing and sustaining cultural safety programs in nursing education and practice. As a former dean of a nursing school, she has worked in partnership with Maori nurse educators to develop undergraduate and postgraduate programs for indigenous students. In June 1995 she was Helen Denne Schulte Visiting Professor at the University of Wisconsin–Madison School of Nursing, where she presented a paper on developing and implementing a bicultural curriculum. Her current research uses life story as a method of inquiry into the lived experiences of nurse educators who teach for social change.

Sharon L. Sims is Professor and Chair of the Family Health Nursing Department at the Indiana University School of Nursing. She is a certified Pediatric Nurse Practitioner and maintains a clinical practice in child health. She has conducted studies in family caregiving and home healthcare, and was instrumental in designing and implementing the narrative-centered Family Nurse Practitioner curriculum at IU. Her current research focuses on "being new" in the nurse practitioner role. She is also a captain in the United States Naval Reserve Nurse Corps.

Jan D. Sinnott is a Professor of Psychology at Towson University in Baltimore, Maryland, where she has taught since 1978. She has worked to bridge the worlds of teaching, research, and clinical practice since her experiences as a postdoctoral fellow and guest scientist at the National Institutes of Health and her work with businesses and government as a consultant. She is author of more than 100 publications, including a dozen books based on her decades of research to create her theory of the development of Complex Postformal Thought. Her latest scholarly books are *The Development of Logic in Adulthood: Postformal Thought and Its Applications* (New York: Plenum/Kluwer, 1998), *Reinventing the University: A Radical Proposal for a Problem-Focused University* (with Lynn Johnson; Ablex, now Elsevier-Holland, 1996), and *The Interdisciplinary Handbook of Adult Lifespan Learning* (Westport, CT: Greenwood, 1994). She has been interviewed by many popular publications, such as *Newsweek* and the *Washington Post*. She is currently working on three books: "Methods for Teaching Complex Postformal Thought in the College Classroom," "Feelings of Community and Adult Development," and "Spirituality and Adult Development." Her current research is focused on methods for the creation of community in the college classroom and students' connection between feeling part of a community and development of Complex Postformal Thought.

Melinda M. Swenson is Associate Professor of Nursing and Coordinator of the Family Nurse Practitioner major at Indiana University School of Nursing in Indianapolis. A certified Family Nurse Practitioner, she has taught advanced practice nursing for more than 20 years. She conducts her own research and supervises graduate students using nontraditional methodologies, especially qualitative description, naturalistic inquiry, hermeneutics, and phenomenology. In 1995, she and Dr. Sharon L. Sims developed the Narrative-Centered Curriculum, currently in use at Indiana University. She has presented this curriculum nationally and internationally, highlighting modifications of Practice-Based Learning, engaged listening, reflective practices, and other new pedagogies. In 2001, she received the Award for Excellence in Teaching from the National League for Nursing.

Index

Interpretive Studies in Healthcare and the Human Sciences

Series Editor
Nancy L. Diekelmann, PhD, RN, FAAN, Helen Denne Schulte Professor, School of Nursing, University of Wisconsin–Madison

Series Associate Editor
Pamela M. Ironside, PhD, RN, Associate Professor, Department of Nursing and Health, Clarke College

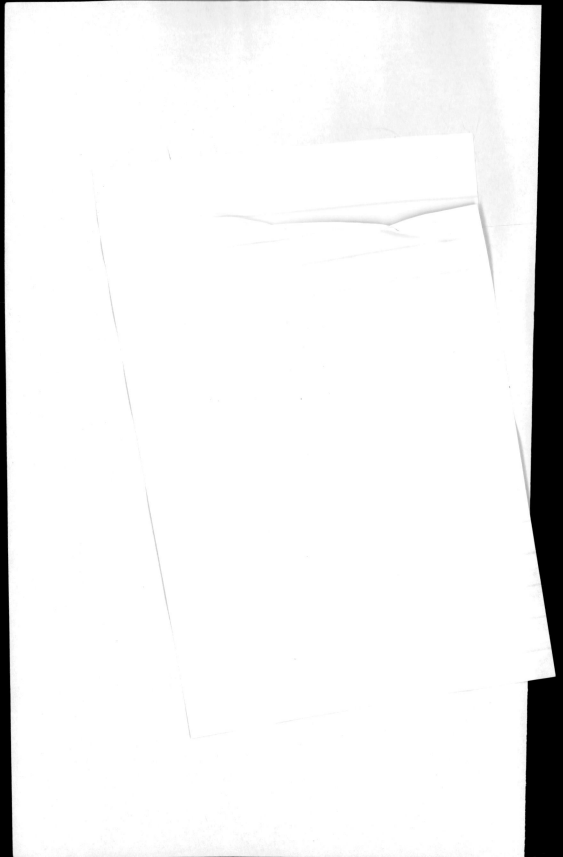